MATERNAL HEALTH
NURSING
REVIEW

SECOND EDITION

Josephine Evans Sagebeer, R.N., C.N.M., M.S.
Clinical Nurse

Department of Clinical Affairs
Plymouth Center for Human Development
Northville, Michigan

ARCO PUBLISHING, INC.
NEW YORK

Second Edition, First Printing, 1979

Published by Arco Publishing, Inc.
219 Park Avenue South, New York, N.Y. 10003

Copyright © 1975, 1979 by Arco Publishing, Inc.

Library of Congress Cataloging in Publication Data

Sagebeer, Josephine Evans.
Maternal health nursing review.

(Arco nursing review series)
Bibliography: p. *viii*
1. Obstetrical nursing—Examinations, questions, etc. I. Title.
RG951.S23 1979   610.73'678   79-1161
ISBN 0-668-04822-0

Printed in the United States of America

Contents

Preface

This book is written for all students of nursing who have an interest in maternal health. Although it is intended primarily as a review book for examinations, many readers will find it helpful in clarifying basic factual information that arises during theoretical lectures or clinical practice sessions in maternity nursing courses.

I have enjoyed writing this book. It has offered me the opportunity to rediscover basic maternity nursing through the writings of others who also share my enthusiasm and interest in this particular field.

I am indebted to those who have helped in making this book possible. Particular thanks are extended to the Maternity Nursing students at The Pennsylvania State University and to the medical and nursing staff on the Maternity Unit, Centre County Community Hospital — Mountainview Unit.

A special note of gratitude is extended to Christine Bartz, whose research assistance throughout the writing of this book was invaluable.

Publisher's Note

In 1977 the World Health Organization recommended the adoption of the Système International d'Unités (SI) by the medical community throughout the world. In this edition, therefore, SI units have been used even though we realize that many of the reference works cited still employ the old system. The changeover to the use of SI units in medicine has been taking place in fragmented fashion, however, and the book reflects this dualism: questions involving feet and inches or pounds and ounces have not been translated, but quantities expressed "per 100 ml" have been changed to "per dL." We hope, though, that the efforts we have made to conform to the new SI unit system will help hasten a conversion that is, in any case, inevitable.

References

Below is a numbered list of reference books pertaining to the material in this book.

On the last line of each test item at the right-hand side appears a number combination that identifies the reference source and the page or pages where the information relating to the question and the correct answer may be found. The first number refers to the textbook in the list and the second number refers to the page of that textbook.

For example: (4:210) is a reference to the fourth book on the list, page 210 of Reeder's *Maternity Nursing*.

1. Alexander, M.M., and Brown, M.S. *Pediatric Physical Diagnosis for Nurses,* McGraw-Hill, New York, 1974.

2. Broadribb, V., and Corliss, C. *Maternal-Child Nursing,* Lippincott, Philadelphia, 1973.

3. Clausen, J.P., et al. *Maternity Nursing Today,* second edition, McGraw-Hill, New York, 1977.

4. Reeder, E., et al. *Maternity Nursing,* thirteenth edition, Lippincott, Philadelphia, 1976.

5. Iorio, J. *Childbirth: Family-Centered Nursing,* third edition, Mosby, St. Louis, 1975.

6. Lerch, C. *Maternity Nursing,* third edition, Mosby, St. Louis, 1978.

7. Lipkin, G. *Parent-Child Nursing: Psychosocial Aspects,* second edition, Mosby, St. Louis, 1978.

8. Ziegel, E., and Conant Van Blarcom, C. *Obstetric Nursing,* sixth edition, Macmillan, New York, 1972.

CHAPTER 1

General Information

It is essential to lay a firm foundation in maternal health nursing so that nurse-practitioners will be able to understand certain critical issues.

A portion of this chapter is devoted to vital statistics that vividly illustrate the facts regarding maternal and child health in the United States. Included here also are questions on abortion, illegitimacy, nurse-midwifery, and family planning. Equally important to the nurse-practitioner is the broad area of education for childbearing and childrearing. Questions in this area are concerned with natural childbirth and group discussion methods in the antepartal and postpartal period.

Comprehension of the material presented in this chapter will add greater understanding to the practice of nursing.

Directions. Each of the questions or incomplete statements below is followed by four suggested answers or completions. Select the BEST answer in each case.

1. The word "obstetrics" is derived from the term "obstetrix," which means

   A. to deliver
   B. midwife
   C. to provide care to
   D. to support   (4:4)

2. Who is given credit for establishing the first lying-in hospital in the United States?

   A. Hunter
   B. Shippen
   C. Peter Chamberlen
   D. Simpson   (4:661)

3. What organization was responsible for conducting the first extensive work in organized prenatal care?

   A. The National Committee for Maternal Health
   B. Maternity Center Association
   C. Children's Bureau
   D. none of the above   (4:665)

4. The United States Children's Bureau was established in

   A. 1900
   B. 1912
   C. 1925
   D. 1932   (4:664)

5. Of the following, who was an early advocate of antenatal care as a necessary part of obstetrics?

   A. Charles White
   B. Oliver Holmes
   C. John William Ballantyne
   D. none of the above   (6:499)

6. What is the name of the woman who provided nursing care to the people in the mountains of North Carolina and for whom an association was named?

   A. Lydia Holman
   B. Mary Breckinridge
   C. Gertrude Kipp
   D. none of the above   (8:786)

7. The World Health Organization was created in

   A. 1930
   B. 1937

C. 1940
D. 1946 (4:666)

8. Antepartal care was *first* provided to women in which of the following cities?

    A. New York City
    B. Boston, Massachusetts
    C. Philadelphia, Pennsylvania
    D. Brooklyn, New York (4:12)

9. Which of the following men first described phenylketonuria?

    A. Hecht
    B. Folling
    C. Jervis
    D. O'Brien (3:211)

10. PKU testing first became mandatory on the state level in

    A. 1950
    B. 1965
    C. 1969
    D. 1970 (4:667)

11. Maternal and child health nursing means

    A. a combination of the traditional courses in maternity and pediatric nursing
    B. a concept of nursing care that takes into consideration the relationship of the mother to the care of her child
    C. the care of healthy mothers and children
    D. all of the above (4:6)

12. Which of the following factors determine(s) the rate at which population grows?

    A. births
    B. deaths
    C. migration
    D. all of the above (4:10)

13. The average-sized family has how many children?

    A. one or two
    B. two or three
    C. three or four
    D. four or five (5:433)

14. The Third White House conference in 1930 focused on which of the following topics?

    A. children in general
    B. all aspects of maternal and child care
    C. children and youth
    D. the dependent child (4:666)

15. What was the name of the doctor who administered chloroform to Queen Victoria for delivery of her child in 1853?

    A. Simpson
    B. Meigs
    C. Snow
    D. Leopold (4:662)

16. The first authentic cesarean section performed on a living mother is credited to

    A. Nufer
    B. Crere
    C. Trautman
    D. none of the above (4:659)

17. Who wrote *System einer vollstandigen medicinischen Polezey?*

    A. John Clarke
    B. Johan Peter Frank
    C. Jakob Kolletschka
    D. none of the above (4:660)

18. Who named the pelvimeter, which is used in obstetrical practice?

    A. Baudeloeque
    B. Johnston
    C. Dare
    D. Smith (4:661)

19. The Birth Registration Area was established as a federal act in

    A. 1910
    B. 1915
    C. 1917
    D. 1920 (4:664)

20. Which of the following nurses was indirectly responsible for the law requiring all physicians and midwives to use prophylaxes in the eyes of the newborn?

    A. Ernestine Wiedenbach
    B. Carolyn Van Blarcom
    C. Erna Ziegel
    D. none of the above (4:664-5)

21. Which famous museum has been reproducing the Dickinson-Belskie models since 1945?

    A. Metropolitan Museum
    B. Field Museum
    C. Cleveland Health Museum
    D. none of the above (4:666)

22. The marriage rate is defined as the number of marriages per

    A. 1,000 population

B. 10,000 population
C. 100,000 population
D. none of the above   (4:8)

23. The fertility rate is the number of births per

A. 1,000 women 15 to 44 years old
B. 10,000 women 19 to 27 years old
C. 1,000 women 19 to 27 years old
D. 10,000 women 15 to 44 years old   (4:8)

24. Maternal mortality is defined as

A. any maternal death during the labor and delivery experience
B. any maternal death during the antepartal, intrapartal, or postpartal experience
C. any maternal death resulting from complications of antepartal, intrapartal, or postpartal experience
D. any maternal death resulting from intrapartal experience and complications of antepartal, intrapartal, and postpartal experience   (2:43)

25. As a result of the rapid reduction in maternal mortality since 1960, the rate of computation for maternal mortality rates

A. is now based on 1,000 live births
B. is now based on 10,000 live births
C. is now based on 100,000 live births
D. none of the above   (3:110)

26. The highest maternal mortality rate occurs in which of the following age groups?

A. 15 to 25
B. 20 to 30
C. 25 to 35
D. over 35   (4:11)

27. There were how many maternal deaths in 1970 based on 100,000 live births?

A. 15.2
B. 18.8
C. 21.5
D. 22.2   (3:111)

28. The number of maternal deaths in 1973 was

A. 200
B. 600
C. 477
D. 700   (3:110)

29. The deceased number of maternal deaths is largely due to improved care during

A. the prenatal period
B. labor and delivery

C. the postpartum period
D. all of the above   (8:772)

30. Generally speaking, the lowest maternal mortality rate occurs in the

A. 10- to 20-year-old range
B. 20- to 30-year-old range
C. 30- to 40-year-old range
D. none of the above   (5:434)

31. The reduction in maternal mortality is the result of

A. more hospital deliveries
B. better use and availability of blood
C. development and use of antibacterial drugs
D. all of the above   (5:434)

32. The most frequent causes of maternal mortality in the United States today are

A. toxemia and medical complications of pregnancy
B. hemorrhage and toxemia
C. hemorrhage and infection
D. abortion and toxemia   (5:434)

33. The total rate of maternal deaths caused by toxemia in the white population is about what percentage per 100,000 live births?

A. 2.2
B. 8.7
C. 15.4
D. 20.0   (3:111)

34. Infant mortality rate means the number of deaths

A. in the first two months of life per 1,000 live births
B. in the first six months of life per 1,000 live births
C. in the first twelve months of life per 1,000 live births
D. none of the above   (3:111)

35. The perinatal period is defined as

A. the week before and the week after delivery
B. the period after the twentieth week of gestation through the twenty-eighth day after birth
C. the period from the twenty-eighth week of gestation through seven days after birth
D. from conception to 28 days after birth   (8:775)

36. Neonatal death rate refers to
    A. deaths among infants (or fetuses) weighing over 500 g per 1,000 live births
    B. infants of 20 week's gestation or more that die in utero per 1,000 population
    C. deaths among infants in first year of life per 1,000 live births
    D. deaths among infants in the first four weeks of life per 1,000 live births   (4:8)

37. The most frequent cause of infant mortality in the United States today is
    A. respiratory disorders
    B. birth injuries
    C. low birth weight of full-term and premature infants
    D. asphyxia   (2:46)

38. In the United States, the incidence of premature births is approximately
    A. 2% of all births
    B. 6% of all births
    C. 8% of all births
    D. 10% of all births   (8:670)

39. An average preinatal mortality rate in the United States would be
    A. 10% of all deaths
    B. 30% of all deaths
    C. 17% of all deaths
    D. 1% of all deaths   (8:775)

40. The birth rate between 1947 and 1968 in the United States
    A. declined about 8.3
    B. remained about the same
    C. increased about 2.5
    D. none of the above   (3:109−10)

41. The birth rate in the United States in 1970 was approximately
    A. 17.4
    B. 18.0
    C. 14.9
    D. 18.6   (6:29)

42. The total infant mortality in 1973 was
    A. 12.4 per 1,000 live births
    B. 14.6 per 1,000 live births
    C. 17.7 per 1,000 live births
    D. 19.8 per 1,000 live births   (3:111)

43. The infant mortality rate in 1973 for non-white babies was
    A. 11.6
    B. 15.8
    C. 26.2
    D. 29.4   (3:111)

44. The world population growth is attributable to
    A. reduction of mortality rate
    B. increase in number of women of childbearing age
    C. both A and B
    D. neither A nor B   (6:28)

45. In 1960 there were approximately how many illegitimate births to teenagers?
    A. 19,200
    B. 91,700
    C. 61,200
    D. 76,400   (2:666)

46. In 1968 the rate of teenage out-of-wedlock births for both white and nonwhite in the 15-to-19 age group was
    A. 10.2
    B. 15.7
    C. 19.8
    D. 22.2   (4:54)

47. Which of the following statements reflects the correct information regarding statistics for legitimacy recorded in 1968?
    A. the rate is highest among women 15 to 24 years of age
    B. more than half of all births were to white mothers
    C. from 1961 to 1968 the rate of illegitimate births dropped
    D. all of the above   (8:783)

48. What percentage of out-of-wedlock pregnancies in 1968 were to nonwhite mothers?
    A. 35%
    B. 55%
    C. 65%
    D. 75%   (8:783)

49. The ratio of illegitimate live births is about
    A. 70 per 1,000 live births
    B. 82 per 1,000 live births
    C. 97 per 1,000 live births
    D. 99 per 1,000 live births   (8:784)

50. "Unwed mother" is a
    A. medical term
    B. sociolegal designation
    C. psychological term
    D. none of the above   (2:237)

51. The Salvation Army opened their first maternity home in
    A. 1852
    B. 1887
    C. 1903
    D. 1915   (6:223)

52. When an adolescent girl becomes pregnant, it is probably best that
    A. she enter a maternity home when the pregnancy becomes evident
    B. she enter a maternity home for the last six weeks of pregnancy
    C. she remain at home
    D. she stay in a foster home   (5:428)

53. Which of the following factors has contributed to the decrease in the number of maternity homes?
    A. legal abortions
    B. the message of Women's Lib
    C. birth control pills
    D. all of the above   (5:431)

54. Which of the following factors contribute(s) to a higher incidence of toxemia in the pregnant girl under the age of 16?
    A. incomplete uterine development
    B. late, irregular prenatal care
    C. improper diet
    D. all of the above   (5:425)

55. Who wrote *House of Tomorrow?*
    A. Mary Hanes
    B. Jean Thompson
    C. Alcian Smith
    D. Jill Thompson   (2:31)

56. Which agency is well known for its research on unwed fathers?
    A. Vista Del Mar
    B. Children's Bureau
    C. Child Study Association of America
    D. Child Welfare League of America
                                      (5:430)

57. Some authorities believe that the unwed father
    A. should never be told about the child he has fathered
    B. should be allowed to see the child he has fathered
    C. should be told about the child he has fathered but never be allowed to see it
    D. none of the above   (5:430)

58. The unmarried teenager who comes from the low socioeconomic class may experience a poor pregnancy outcome because
    A. she may not be physically up to par
    B. she may be socially deprived
    C. she may be lacking in education
    D. all of the above   (6:225)

59. Among teenage pregnancies there is a high incidence of
    A. cardiac problems in the infant
    B. diabetes in the teenager
    C. prematurity in the infant
    D. all of the above   (2:666)

60. Which of the following complications are commonly found in the adolescent pregnant girl?
    1. anemia
    2. toxemia
    3. pelvic contractures
    4. premature infants
    5. low-birth-weight infants
    A. 2, 3
    B. 2, 4, 5
    C. 1, 3, 5
    D. all of the above   (2:239)

61. The pregnant teenager needs how much calcium daily?
    A. 1.3 g
    B. 1.7 g
    C. 2.0 g
    D. 2.2 g   (8:148)

62. The calcium input can best be insured by asking the adolescent girl to drink how much milk daily over and above the recommended amount?
    A. one glass
    B. three glasses
    C. four glasses
    D. none of the above   (8:148)

63. The pregnant adolescent may have an especially low retention level of
    A. calcium
    B. vitamin C
    C. iron
    D. all of the above   (6:160)

64. The pregnant teenager may have nutritional problems associated with
    A. her phase of normal development
    B. her environment

C. her reaction to the pregnancy itself
D. all of the above   (6:160)

65. The nurse can be most therapeutic to the un-married pregnant teenager by

A. helping her with the psychological pro-blems that may have caused the preg-nancy
B. helping her make the decision as to keeping or giving up her child for adop-tion
C. being a good listener
D. none of the above   (6:226)

66. During the labor and delivery process the unwed mother

A. needs the same kind of nursing care as any other mother
B. should be left alone except when necessary routines must be performed
C. needs more support than the married mother
D. should be encouraged to bring her mother with her   (5:429)

67. Which of the following statements *best* describes the reaction of the unwed mother toward her child if there are abnormalities present at birth?

A. she will become morose and withdrawn
B. she will not assume any responsibility for these problems in the child
C. she will question the feasibility of plac-ing this child for adoption
D. she will directly blame herself for the problems in the child   (5:37–8)

68. Which of the following agencies sets the standards for adoptive procedures?

A. Child Study Association of America
B. Children's Bureau
C. Child Welfare League of America
D. none of these   (2:34)

69. The girl who plans to give her child up for adoption

A. should not be allowed to see her baby because she might change her mind
B. should be told the sex of the child and other information she might ask re-garding the infant, but should not see the child
C. should be permitted to see and provide care for her child if she so wishes
D. should be forced to see and hold the baby   (2:36)

70. What percentage of families today is headed by a woman rather than the traditional man?

A. 2%
B. 4%
C. 8%
D. 10%   (3:100)

71. In 1970 approximately what percentage of women in the United States held full-time positions outside the home?

A. 10%
B. 15%
C. 25%
D. 40%   (3:104)

72. The changes in the family life style in the United States have most widely resulted in

A. more women giving up their out-of-wedlock babies for adoption
B. increasing numbers of women who marry the father of their illegitimately conceived child so that the infant can be raisedin a two-parent family
C. more women who keep and raise their children in a single-parent setting
D. increasing numbers of women who are able to adopt illegitimate babies (3:103)

73. The sexually active teenager should

A. have access to the most effective methods of contraception
B. be referred to a mental health clinic for therapy
C. be denied any method of family plan-ning
D. none of the above   (3:223)

74. The use of contraceptive pills for the teenager has been most highly questioned for which of the following reasons?

A. it may cause increased sexual activity
B. it may cause retardation of the growth of the teenagers' bones
C. it may cause psychological problems
D. none of these   (6:46)

75. Conventional family planning programs do not always assist in preventing pregnancies in the adolescent population because

A. contraceptives are not always available to the sexually active teenager until after a pregnancy has occurred
B. teenagers admit that they had not ex-pected to become involved in inter-course with their partners

C. the taking of contraceptives in itself is an admission of the intent to have sexual relations
D. all of these   (7:20−1)

76. The ideal age for reproduction appears to be
    A. below the age of 20 years
    B. between the ages of 20 and 25 years
    C. between the ages of 25 and 30 years
    D. between the ages of 30 and 35 years
                                    (6:21)

77. The first birth control center in the United States was opened in
    A. 1912
    B. 1916
    C. 1920
    D. 1925   (6:20)

78. The founder of the Planned Parenthood Federation of America was
    A. Margaret Sanger
    B. Louis Hellman
    C. Duncan Reed
    D. none of the above   (6:20)

79. Planned Parenthood−World Population was established in
    A. 1950
    B. 1955
    C. 1960
    D. 1965   (6:20)

80. In what year was the Margaret Sanger Research Bureau established?
    A. 1915
    B. 1918
    C. 1921
    D. 1923   (4:666)

81. The diaphragm was first introduced in
    A. 1912
    B. 1918
    C. 1924
    D. none of the above   (6:34)

82. The percentage of patients in planned parenthood clinics who choose a diaphragm as a contraceptive method is about
    A. 1%
    B. 5%
    C. 10%
    D. 15%   (3:242)

83. The correct use of a diaphragm as a contraceptive method results in approximately how many pregnancies per year?
    A. no pregnancies per 100 women
    B. 3 pregnancies per 100 women
    C. 10 pregnancies per 100 women
    D. none of the above   (3:242)

84. The diaphragm should be left in place for how long following coitus?
    A. about one hour
    B. about two hours
    C. about four hours
    D. about six hours   (6:36)

85. The chief objection to the diaphragm as a contraceptive by its users is
    A. it is uncomfortable for the man
    B. it is uncomfortable for the woman
    C. it requires vaginal manipulation in order to insert it properly
    D. it can cause pelvic inflammatory disease   (2:227)

86. The primary function of the diaphragm is
    A. to act as a mechanical barrier to the entry of the sperm
    B. to hold the spermicidal jelly or cream
    C. to provide a pouch where negative pressure will be present
    D. none of the above   (3:241)

87. The first hormonal contraceptives were introduced in the United States in
    A. 1950
    B. 1955
    C. 1960
    D. 1965   (6:28)

88. Which of the following types of birth control first suppresses the follicle-stimulating hormone and then both the follicle-stimulating and luteinizing hormones?
    A. oral contraceptive −combined type
    B. oral contraceptive −sequential type
    C. both A and B
    D. neither A nor B   (6:30)

89. Approximately how many different types of oral contraceptives are available in the United States?
    A. 10
    B. 15
    C. 20
    D. none of the above   (6:28)

90. What percentage of women who discontinue the use of an oral contraceptive will both menstruate and ovulate in their first postpill cycle?
    A. 15%
    B. 25%
    C. 50%
    D. 90%   (6:30)

91. The woman who is taking oral contraceptive pills should be advised to report which of the following symptoms to her doctor?
    1. frequent headaches
    2. persistent headaches
    3. sudden edema
    4. pronounced pain in her legs

    A. 1, 3, 4
    B. 2, 3, 4
    C. none of these
    D. all of these   (6:31)

92. Which of the following is the commonly accepted reason for nausea and vomiting while taking the oral contraceptive pill?
    A. progestogen causes irritation of the gastrointestinal lining
    B. estrogen is a gastrointestinal irritant
    C. there are psychological implications to taking the birth control pill
    D. none of the above   (6:31)

93. The preferred time for insertion of an IUD is
    A. immediately before the menstrual period
    B. during the first two days of the menstrual period
    C. during the last few days of the menstrual period
    D. midway between menstrual periods
                                    (3:238-9)

94. Which of the following symptoms are considered to be side effects associated with the IUD?
    1. regulation of menstrual cycle
    2. decrease in menstrual flow
    3. reduction of dysmenorrhea
    4. premenstrual tension
    5. vaginal discharge

    A. 1, 2, 3
    B. 4, 5
    C. all of the above
    D. none of the above   (3:239-40)

95. The failure rate for women who retain an IUD is about
    A. 0.5% during the first year
    B. 2% during the first year
    C. 5% during the first year
    D. 8% during the first year   (3:239)

96. Intrauterine contraceptive devices prevent pregnancy by
    A. altering the environment in the fallopian tubes
    B. altering the environment in the endometrium
    C. changing the traveling speed of the ovum
    D. action not exactly known   (8:502)

97. The nylon tab attached to the end of the IUD that extends from the vaginal canal is called the
    A. string
    B. tab
    C. cervical appendage
    D. none of the above   (6:36)

98. A method whereby temporary abstinence is practiced during the fertile period of the menstrual cycle is
    A. foaming tablets method
    B. coitus interruptus method
    C. rhythm method
    D. none of the above   (8:495)

99. In utilizing the rhythm method, the period during which a woman may conceive extends through
    A. the day of the temperature rise
    B. one day after the temperature drop
    C. two days after the temperature drop
    D. three days after the temperature drop
                                    (4:127)

100. Failure in contraceptive control while using the rhythm method can occur when
    A. the menses are irregular
    B. there is early unexpected ovulation
    C. there is delayed ovulation
    D. all of the above   (6:49)

101. The rhythm method is also referred to as
    1. periodic continence
    2. coitus interruptus
    3. temporary abstinence
    4. postcoital douche
    5. safe period

    A. 2, 4

B. 1, 3, 5
C. 3, 5
D. none of the above   (3:245)

102. Coitus interruptus is a method of birth control whereby

A. the sperm are not produced
B. the sperm are of such a low count that conception cannot take place
C. the sperm are not deposited in the vagina
D. the sperm are deposited in the vagina during the safe period   (8:494)

103. Generally speaking, coitus interruptus is not considered to be a satisfactory method of birth control because

A. it limits full sexual gratification
B. it demands a great deal of trust on the part of the woman
C. there is pre-ejaculatory secretion
D. all of the above   (4:128)

104. The condom was introduced primarily as a means to avoid

A. venereal infection
B. conception
C. both A and B
D. neither A nor B   (6:34)

105. Another name for the condom is

A. prophylactic
B. rubber
C. safes
D. all of the above   (8:499)

106. The correct use of the condom results in what percentage of accidental pregnancies per year?

A. 0.05%
B. 1%
C. 3%
D. none of the above   (3:246)

107. When spermicidal preparations are used to prevent pregnancy, at which point following coitus may a douche be taken without increasing the risk of pregnancy?

A. immediately after coitus
B. three hours after coitus
C. five hours after coitus
D. six hours after coitus   (6:34)

108. When spermicidal preparations are used they should be inserted

A. within three hours before coitus
B. within two hours before coitus

C. within one hour before coitus
D. none of these   (6:34)

109. Approximately how much time should elapse between insertion of a vaginal suppository and intercourse?

A. 5 minutes
B. 10 minutes
C. 30 minutes
D. none of these   (3:247)

110. How much time should elapse between insertion of a foaming tablet and coitus?

A. 5 minutes
B. 10 minutes
C. 15 minutes
D. no need to wait any amount of time   (3:247)

111. Generally speaking, which method of conception control appears to be preferred by the American woman?

A. pill
B. IUD
C. rhythm
D. diaphragm   (3:237)

112. Which of the following would be considered the *least* dependable method of contraception?

A. rhythm method
B. intrauterine device
C. postcoital douche
D. spermicidal jelly or cream   (8:494)

113. Which of the following should *not* be left in place during the entire menstrual period?

A. diaphragm
B. cervical lays
C. IUD
D. all of these can be left in place during the entire menstrual cycle   (6:36)

114. The most effective method of contraception at present is

A. rhythm
B. oral hormones
C. diaphragm
D. vaginal cream or suppositories   (2:225)

115. Excessive mucus secretion from the vaginal canal can be used as an indication of ovulation during which of the following methods of birth control?

A. oral contraceptive —combined type
B. oral contraceptive —sequential type

C. rhythm method
D. IUD   (6:49)

116. The purpose of the Sims-Huhner test is

A. to determine whether the fallopian tubes are open
B. to determine sperm survival and motility
C. to test for ovulation
D. none of these   (3:164)

117. A vasectomy takes approximately

A. 10 to 15 minutes
B. 20 to 30 minutes
C. 30 to 40 minutes
D. none of these   (6:51)

118. Male sterilization is considered to be reversible in what percent of cases?

A. 5 to 10%
B. 10 to 20%
C. 20 to 40%
D. it is not reversible   (3:244)

119. The man who has been sterilized should be told

A. that his body is no longer capable of producing sperm
B. that he is capable of fertilizing an ovum for about four ejaculations
C. that his sperm will remain viable for about ten more ejaculations
D. that he will no longer have ejaculations   (3:244)

120. Which state in the union was the first to pass an abortion law?

A. Massachusetts
B. Connecticut
C. New York
D. New Jersey   (3:173)

121. Who was the London surgeon who was responsible for the first decisive move in abortion reform?

A. John Snow
B. Aleck Bourne
C. Donald Harting
D. none of these   (3:174)

122. In 1970 the largest number of legal abortions were obtained by women in which of the following age groups?

A. 15 to 24 years
B. 25 to 32 years
C. 33 to 42 years
D. none of these   (3:178)

123. In 1970 the largest number of legal abortions were done during which of the following time periods?

A. 1 to 9 weeks
B. 9 to 12 weeks
C. 13 to 16 weeks
D. 17 to 20 weeks   (3:180)

124. Tubal ligation in women should be done preferably

A. right after a spontaneous abortion
B. following the six-week check
C. when the last child is about six months old
D. during the immediate post-delivery period   (3:244)

125. Which of the following procedures are associated with laparoscopic tubal sterilization?

1. Falope ring
2. puncture of cul-de-sac
3. spring-loaded clip
4. electrocoagulation
5. incision of ductus deferens

A. 1, 2, 3
B. 1, 3, 4
C. 2, 5
D. all of the above   (6:50—1)

126. The hazard associated with a laparoscopic sterlization is

A. carbon monoxide embolism
B. carbon dioxide embolism
C. failure to obtain permanent sterilization
D. all of these   (6:50)

127. In what year did the United States Supreme Court decree that the decision to seek an abortion during the first trimester of pregnancy was entirely between the woman and her doctor?

A. 1965
B. 1968
C. 1970
D. none of these   (6:55)

128. Which of the following types of abortion is usually done immediately after the woman misses a period?

A. dilatation and curettage
B. dilatation and vacuum aspiration
C. pre-emptive abortion
D. saline amnioinfusion   (6:60)

129. Which of the following methods of abortion has been known to increase the number of fetal erythrocytes in the mother's blood?
    A. dilatation and curettage
    B. dilatation and vacuum aspiration
    C. pre-emptive amnion fusion
    D. none of the above   (6:38)

130. What is the name given to the fatty acid extract in human seminal fluid that causes myometrial tissue to contract and relax?
    A. proteolytic enzymes
    B. prostaglandin
    C. semen
    D. testosterone   (6:61)

131. Who named this fatty acid extract in the human seminal fluid?
    A. Ulf Svante von Euler
    B. Oscar Harkavy
    C. F.E. Rubocitis
    D. J.R. Zabriskie   (6:61)

132. Who discovered that a high concentration of two of the prostaglandins circulate through the venous blood of women during labor?
    A. S.M. Karim
    B. G.M. Filshie
    C. Christopher Tietze
    D. none of the above   (6:61)

133. Which of the following symptoms are the result of excessive progestogens in the body?
    1. tenderness in the breasts
    2. increased appetite
    3. candidal vaginitis
    4. weight gain
    5. fatigue
    A. 1, 4
    B. 2, 3, 5
    C. 1, 3, 4, 5
    D. none of these   (6:30)

134. Which of the following are considered to be side effects of prostaglandins while being administered via the intravenous route?
    1. nausea
    2. heavy show
    3. high blood pressure
    4. excessive cramping
    5. diarrhea
    A. 1, 2, 3
    B. 1, 5
    C. none of these
    D. all of these   (6:62)

135. In 1973 the largest number of abortions were obtained by women between the ages of
    A. 14 and 18
    B. 15 and 24
    C. 20 and 28
    D. none of the above   (3:178)

136. In 1970 the most frequently used procedure for induced abortion was
    A. D and C
    B. D and E
    C. saline induction
    D. hysterectomy   (3:180)

137. Following saline infusion into the uterine cavity, spontaneous labor starts
    A. immediately
    B. within 10 hours
    C. between 12 and 36 hours
    D. none of the above   (3:183)

138. In a saline induction fetal death can occur
    A. within 15 minutes
    B. within 30 minutes
    C. within 60 minutes
    D. none of the above   (3:192)

139. In performing a saline amnioinfusion, what percentage of hypertonic saline solution is used?
    A. 10%
    B. 20%
    C. 30%
    D. none of these   (6:60)

140. Which of the following are considered to be complications associated with saline amnioinfusion?
    A. excessive bleeding
    B. fever
    C. bacteremia
    D. all of these   (6:62)

141. It is usually recommended that a dilatation and curettage be performed on a primigravida before the
    A. eighth week of gestation
    B. tenth week of gestation
    C. twelfth week of gestation
    D. sixth week of gestation   (6:59)

142. Which of the following abortive procedures may be safely used on a woman who is more than 12 weeks pregnant?
    A. dilation and vacuum aspiration
    B. pre-emptive abortion

C. saline amnioinfusion
D. none of these　　　　　(6:60)

143. What is the approximate percentage of complications in women who have early abortions?

    A. 1%
    B. 2%
    C. 5%
    D. 10%　　　　　(6:62)

144. Which of the following complications can result from abortions?

    1. infections
    2. uterine perforations
    3. uterine hemorrhage
    4. cervical lacerations
    5. chronic menstrual problems

    A. 1, 2, 3
    B. 2, 3, 4, 5
    C. none of the above
    D. all of the above　　　　　(6:62)

145. What is the approximate percentage of complications in women who have late abortions?

    A. 5%
    B. 10%
    C. 20%
    D. 30%　　　　　(6:62)

146. Who first used the term "natural childbirth" in reference to a type of childbirth in which the woman was an active participant in the total process?

    A. Fernand Lamaze
    B. Elizabeth Bing
    C. Erna Wright
    D. Grantly Dick Read　　　　　(8:788)

147. Which of the following organizations was established to promote the learning method of preparation for childbirth education in the United States?

    A. Childbirth Education Association
    B. American Society for Psychoprophylaxis in Obstetrics
    C. Maternity Center Association
    D. LaLeche League　　　　　(8:790)

148. Which of the following was (were) responsible for introducing the Read Method to the people of the United States?

    1. Grace—New Haven Community Hospital
    2. Yale University School of Medicine
    3. Yale University School of Nursing
    4. Boston Hospital for Women

    A. 1, 3, 4
    B. 1, 2, 4, 5
    C. 1, 2, 3, 4
    D. 4, 5　　　　　(8:785)

149. The International Childbirth Education Association was founded in

    A. 1940
    B. 1950
    C. 1960
    D. 1970　　　　　(2:34)

150. Who originated the concept that pain during labor was caused by fear?

    A. Clement Yahia
    B. Grantly Dick Read
    C. Fernand Lamaze
    D. Helen Heardman　　　　　(8:165)

151. Which school of thought believes that stimulus-response conditioning during pregnancy will eliminate the pain associated with childbirth?

    A. hypnosis
    B. the Read method
    C. psychoprophylactic method
    D. husband-coached method　　　　　(3:373)

152. Psychoprophylactic childbirth became popular in the United States mainly through the efforts of

    A. Dr. Thomas
    B. the LaLeche League
    C. Marjorie Karmel
    D. Elizabeth Bing　　　　　(4:224)

153. The psychoprophylactic method was first used where in the United States?

    A. Hartford, Connecticut
    B. Boston, Massachusetts
    C. New Haven, Connecticut
    D. Springfield, Massachusetts　　　　　(8:789)

154. Who of the following were the *first* to actively support psychoprophylactic childbirth?

    1. Nicolaiev
    2. Bulganin
    3. Velvovskiy
    4. Simonov
    5. Stoianavich

    A. 1, 3
    B. 1, 2, 3
    C. 2, 4, 5
    D. all of the above　　　　　(4:224)

155. The psychoprophylactic method of natural childbirth was *first* started in

    A. France
    B. England
    C. Russia
    D. the United States   (4:224)

156. Who proved the theory that reaction to a stimulus could be learned by training?

    A. Grantly Dick Read
    B. Fernand Lamaze
    C. Ivan Pavlov
    D. Pierre Valley   (7:75)

157. The Lamaze method of natural childbirth should ideally be taught to the pregnant woman and her husband at about the

    A. sixth week of pregnancy
    B. twenty-second week of pregnancy
    C. twenty-eighth week of pregnancy
    D. thirty-fourth week of pregnancy (7:76)

158. The goal of the Lamaze natural childbirth method is to prepare women

    A. for a painless childbirth through controlled breathing and relaxation
    B. to control the amount of discomfort which results from the labor and delivery process
    C. to deliver her baby vaginally without the aid of medications
    D. none of the above   (7:76)

159. Motherliness can be thought of as

    A. the enactment of the role of mother, involving skills and having a certain understanding of the developmental process of the child
    B. an emotional feeling that develops with time as the mother has increasing contact with her infant
    C. the anticipated role of a woman as she looks forward to childbirth and childbearing
    D. none of the above   (4:20)

160. The Maternity Center Association approach to preparation for childbirth is based on principles of

    A. hypnosis
    B. relaxation
    C. pain
    D. culturally determined factors (4:225)

161. Group health teaching should be based on which of the following points?

    1. parents can learn from each other
    2. each parent learns in his own way
    3. parents learn best what they want to learn
    4. parents can learn

    A. 1, 2
    B. 3, 4
    C. 1, 2, 3
    D. all of the above   (3:129−30)

162. In the group discussion method of education, the leader serves in the role of

    A. authority person
    B. observer
    C. resource persons
    D. secretary   (3:129)

163. In the group discussion methods, the leader ideally

    A. presents the topics for discussion
    B. sets the atmosphere for a question-answer type of interaction
    C. guides the discussion and opens up essential areas not covered by the group
    D. all of the above   (4:222)

164. Education for expectant parents should

    A. include aspects relating to childbearing
    B. stress information regarding pregnancy, labor and delivery, and postpartum care
    C. be broadly based in scope and include issues beyond the pregnancy cycle itself
    D. look at care for both mother and child throughout the entire cycle (3:153)

165. The LaLeche League was organized in

    A. 1950
    B. 1956
    C. 1962
    D. 1966   (5:436)

166. Which of the following is one of the main goals of the LaLeche League?

    A. to assist women who are planning to have natural childbirth
    B. to support and encourage women who are breast feeding their infants
    C. to provide help for Spanish-speaking women during their confinement
    D. all of the above   (2:33)

167. Abdominal breathing is done during labor primarily to
    A. equalize pressure between the abdominal cavity and the uterine cavity
    B. help women maintain control
    C. lift up the abdominal wall from the uterus
    D. provide distraction for women   (2:91)

168. Tailor sitting during pregnancy accomplishes which of the following purposes?
    A. provides relaxation of the inner thigh muscles
    B. helps stretch the thigh and pelvic floor muscles
    C. helps relieve backache
    D. all of the above   (2:93)

169. What organization during the early 1940s was responsible for originating the concept of "rooming in"?
    A. International Childbirth Education Association
    B. Cornelian Corner
    C. LaLeche League
    D. Children's Bureau   (8:791)

170. Which explanation given by the nurse would best explain the concept of "rooming in"? It is an arrangement whereby
    A. the mother and baby are together and the mother assumes complete care of her baby
    B. the mother and her newborn are cared for together in the same hospital unit
    C. the mother is able to have the baby brought to her whenever she desires
    D. the mother can best meet all of the infant's needs throughout the hospital stay   (8:751)

171. One of the earliest books written for the expectant woman was
    A. The Prospective Mother
    B. Prenatal Care
    C. The Womanly Art of Breast Feeding
    D. Thank You, Dr. Lamaze   (8:781)

172. Who is responsible for publishing the popular pamphlets entitled Prenatal Care and Infant Care?
    A. Department of Health, Education and Welfare
    B. Children's Bureau
    C. International Childbirth Education Association
    D. none of the above   (8:781)

173. The purpose(s) of exercises in a childbirth education program is (are) to
    1. promote comfort during pregnancy
    2. facilitate childbirth
    3. provide diversion during pregnancy
    4. aid in strengthening muscles during the puerperium
    A. 1, 3
    B. 1, 2, 3
    C. 1, 2, 4
    D. all of the above   (5:75)

174. During the first trimester of pregnancy the nurse should focus her teaching on the
    A. mother's general health
    B. preparations for labor and delivery
    C. preparations for the new baby
    D. none of the above   (5:74)

175. Instructions during the second trimester of pregnancy should include
    A. exercises for labor and delivery
    B. fetal growth and development
    C. postpartum exercise
    D. all of the above   (5:75)

176. During the third trimester of pregnancy the woman is most ready for instructions regarding
    A. her future role as wife and mother
    B. plans for the baby's layette
    C. labor and delivery
    D. her husband's role as new father   (5:75)

177. Which of the following exercises should be done in the postpartum period only upon the order of the physician?
    A. lying on abdomen
    B. leg-raising exercises
    C. knee-chest position
    D. none of the above   (4:395)

178. The postpartum mother should first be encouraged to attend group classes
    A. during the taking-in phase
    B. during the taking-hold phase
    C. on her day of discharge
    D. following her discharge from the hospital   (4:368)

179. The trained nurse-midwife was first used in the United States in
    A. Massachusetts, 1620
    B. Pennsylvania, 1770
    C. Kentucky, 1925
    D. New Mexico, 1945   (4:636−7)

180. The Maternity Center Association was founded in

    A. 1900
    B. 1918
    C. 1920
    D. 1930   (4:637)

181. A woman's concept of the mother role is based on which of the following factors?

    A. norms of the culture
    B. social class to which she belongs
    C. type of socialization she has received from her family
    D. all of the above   (4:20)

182. The American College of Nurse-Midwifery was established in

    A. 1925
    B. 1935
    C. 1945
    D. 1955   (4:637)

183. The founder of the Frontier Nursing Service was

    A. Hazel Corbin
    B. Mary Breckinridge
    C. Lillian Wald
    D. Carolyn C. van Blarcom   (4:632)

184. The Maternity Center established its school of nurse-midwifery in

    A. 1920
    B. 1927
    C. 1932
    D. 1934   (4:637)

185. The Frontier Graduate School of Midwifery was opened in

    A. 1926
    B. 1929
    C. 1935
    D. 1939   (4:637)

186. Approximately how many nurse-midwifery educational programs are there in the United States?

    A. five
    B. ten
    C. fifteen
    D. twenty   (6:500)

187. The American College of Nurse-Midwifery recognizes that the nurse-midwife is

    A. ultimately responsible for each patient's care
    B. not responsible for any obstetrical care she provides

    C. a practitioner who functions within the framework of a medically directed health service
    D. responsible only for certain nursing aspects of the patient's care   (6:500)

188. In what year did the American College of Nurse-Midwifery become a member of the International Confederation of Midwives?

    A. 1955
    B. 1957
    C. 1961
    D. 1969   (4:637)

189. Which of the following is *not* inherent in the functioning of the nurse-midwife?

    A. evaluation of progress and management of labor and delivery
    B. care of normal mothers during pregnancy
    C. evaluation and care of newborns
    D. none of these   (4:638–9)

190. Who was the first nurse in the United States to register as a midwife?

    A. Vera Keane
    B. Lydia Holman
    C. Carolyn van Blarcom
    D. none of the above   (4:665)

191. The Dominican monk who, in the thirteenth century, wrote a book for the guidance of midwives was

    A. Albertus Magnus
    B. Soranus of Ephesus
    C. Louis Bourgeois
    D. none of the above   (6:499)

192. There is a reference to the midwife in what chapter of the Bible?

    A. Genesis
    B. Exodus
    C. Leviticus
    D. Numbers   (6:499)

193. Which hospital in the United States is given credit for being the first to give instructions in midwifery?

    A. Cook County
    B. Bellevue
    C. Massachusetts General
    D. Boston Lying-In   (6:500)

194. The first male midwife on record in the United States is

    A. Johnson
    B. Attwood

C. Jackson
D. Livingston   (6:500)

195. Who was the man primarily responsible for bringing about physician participation in midwifery?

A. Louis Bourgeois
B. Julian Clement
C. Hendrik van Deventer
D. James Simpson   (6:500)

196. Home deliveries are advantageous for several reasons. Which of the following is *not* true of in-home deliveries?

A. less expensive
B. less danger of infection
C. adequate facilities to conduct the delivery
D. more emotional support from husband and family   (2:21)

197. What percentage of all deliveries were done in the hospital in 1935?

A. 10%
B. 37%
C. 40%
D. 55%   (8:777)

198. What percentage of nonwhite births are being done in the hospital?

A. 75%
B. 85%
C. 94%
D. 99%   (8:777)

Directions: Each group of numbered words or phrases is followed by a list of lettered statements. MATCH the lettered statement with the numbered word or phrase most closely associated with it.

Questions 199 through 202

199. man who described podalic version and made the procedure more practicable
200. man who started using the bed for deliveries and contributed his views on epidemic puerperal fever and pelvic anatomy
201. man who wrote about the mechanism of labor and earned the title "father of modern midwifery"

202. man who wrote a book on midwifery and contributed modern knowledge on the placenta

A. Mauriceau
B. Pare
C. van Deventer
D. Smellie   (6:500)

Questions 203 through 206

203. concerned with the health and welfare of children and mothers
204. concerned with attainment of the highest possible level of health throughout the world
205. provides leadership in instituting and coordinating child and parent programs
206. assistance to the homeless child

A. WHO
B. Children's Bureau
C. UNICEF
D. ISS   (2:37−40)

Questions 207 through 210

207. *Awake and Aware*
208. *A Way to Natural Childbirth*
209. *Revelation of Childbirth*
210. *Parents Learn through Discussion*

A. Grantly Dick Read
B. Alene Auerbach
C. Irwin Chabon
D. Helen Heardman
        (3:129−30, 370−71; 6:23; 8:788−89)

Questions 211 through 214

211. flexion of baby's head with one hand while the child's body is supported with the other hand and arm
212. rotation of baby's head to occiput anterior position
213. pressure on the occipital portion of the baby's head with one hand and pressure on the baby's brow with the other hand
214. palpation of the head and buttocks of the baby

A. Scanzoni maneuver
B. Leopold's maneuver
C. Ritgen's maneuver
D. Mauriceau maneuver
            (8:274, 384, 453, 456)

Answers and Explanations: General Information

1. **B.** The verb form "obsto" means to stand by, and thus the term "obstetrix" originally applied to the woman who stood in attendance during labor and delivery.

2. **B.** Shippen provided convenient lodgings for the accommodation of poor women during their confinement, and this is said to be the first lying-in hospital in America.

3. **B.** The Maternity Center Association is given credit for establishing the first extensive work in organized prenatal care. The date was 1915.

4. **B.** The Children's Bureau was established in 1912.

5. **C.** John William Ballantyne wrote about antenatal pathology and hygiene.

6. **A.** Lydia Holman is remembered for her contributions to maternity and midwifery. The Holman Association was named for her.

7. **D.** The World Health Organization was created in 1946. The purpose of this organization is "the attainment of the highest possible level of health of all the people."

8. **B.** Antepartal care was first provided in 1901 when the Instructive Nursing Association of Boston began to pay visits to women who were in Boston Lying-in Hospital.

9. **B.** PKU was first described by Folling in 1934 and later in 1953; Hervis identified the missing enzyme as phenylalanine hydroxylase.

10. **B.** PKU testing became mandatory for all infants in the states of Illinois and Michigan, thus setting a precedent for other states.

11. **D.** The term "maternal and child health nursing" has a wide variety of meanings, depending on who is using the term.

12. **D.** All of the factors mentioned are important in determining the rate at which the population grows.

13. **A.** Ten years ago the average family had two to four children. Today families are having 1.8 children.

14. **B.** The Third White House Conference in 1930 focused on all aspects of maternal and child care.

15. **C.** Dr. John Snow administered chloroform to Queen Victoria during the delivery of Prince Leopold in 1853.

16. **C.** Trautman is credited with having performed the first cesarean section on a living woman in 1610.

17. **B.** Frank's work is considered even today to be a landmark in the history of thought on the social relations of health and disease.

18. **A.** Baudeloeque also named and described positions and presentations.

19. **B.** At this time the federal government began to collect data regarding births and handle this data in an organized way.

20. **B.** Carolyn van Blarcom was the executive secretary of the National Society for the Prevention of Blindness, through whose investigations it was learned that the greatest cause of blindness was ophthalmia neonatorum.

21. **C.** The Dickinson-Belskie models are a sculptural set of models representing the birth process.

22. **A.** The marriage rate is defined as the number of marriages per 1,000 total population.

23. **A.** The fertility rate is the number of births per 1,000 women aged 15 to 44 years.

24. **C.** Deaths during the childbearing experience must be the direct or indirect result of the pregnancy.

25. **C.** Before 1960 the rate was determined on the basis of 10,000 live births; now it is based on 100,000 live births.

26. **D.** The highest mortality rate occurs in the over-35-year age group.

27. **C.** In 1970 there were 21.5 deaths per 100,000 live births: 14.4 white deaths and 55.9 nonwhite deaths.

28. **C.** The actual number of maternal deaths in 1973 was 477.

29. **A.** At the same time, improved prenatal care has reduced the incidence of toxemia.

30. **B.** During the 20- to 30-year period the outlook is best.

31. **D.** All these factors have contributed to a decrease in maternal mortality.

32. **C.** Anesthesia and embolism rank third before toxemia, which is now the fourth cause of maternal death in the United States.

33. **A.** The total rate of maternal deaths caused by toxemia in the white population is 2.2. However, in the nonwhite population it is about 9.2.

34. **C.** Some statistics, however, express the ratio of these deaths per 10,000 or 100,000.

35. **B.** Slightly different definitions may be used for this term, as a definite standard has not yet been established.

36. **D.** Some statistics express the ratio of these deaths per 10,000 or 100,000.

37. **C.** Also high on the list of causes of deaths to infants are congenital malformations, birth injuries, and respiratory disorders.

38. **C.** Approximately two thirds of all deaths in the first month of life are related to prematurity.

39. **A.** It is anticipated that this figure will drop in the years to come because of improving maternal and child care.

40. **A.** In 1947 the birth rate was at an all-time high of 25.8 per 1,000 population. In 1968 the rate was 17.5 per 1,000 population.

41. **C.** In 1970 the birth rate was 18.2.

42. **C.** The infant mortality rate in 1973 was 17.7 per 1,000 live births.

43. **C.** The infant mortality rate for nonwhite babies in 1973 was 26.2, whereas for white babies it was 15.8.

44. **C.** The world population growth is attributed to success in reducing the mortality rate and also to the increase in the number of women of childbearing age.

45. **B.** In 1960 there were 91,100 illegitimate births to teenage girls, of whom 48,300 were girls of school age.

46. **C.** The rate of teenage out-of-wedlock births in the United States in the 15- to 19-year-old age group increased from 8.3 in 1940 to 19.8 in 1968.

47. **A.** The statistics gathered by the National Vital Statistics Division indicate that the illegitimacy rate is highest among women 15 to 24 years of age.

48. **C.** In 1968 65% of all out-of-wedlock pregnancies were to nonwhite mothers.

49. **C.** The ratio of illegitimate live births has been about 97 per 1,000 total births.

50. **B.** The phrase "unwed mother" is a sociolegal designation.

51. **B.** The Salvation Army opened its first Maternity Home in Brooklyn, New York, during the year 1887.

52. **C.** When the unwed mother remains at home within her own family there is less loss of self-esteem.

53. **D.** All of the factors mentioned have contributed to the decrease in the number of maternity homes.

54. **D.** All of the factors contribute to the higher incidence of toxemia, with a resulting higher incidence of prematurity and fetal and perinatal deaths.

55. **B.** Jean Thompson, in *House of Tomorrow*, writes about her personal experiences while in a maternity home waiting the birth of her own child.

56. **A.** Vista Delmar, which is located in Los Angeles, California, has carried out much research on unwed fathers.

57. **B.** At Vista Delmar, it is believed that the unwed father should be shown his baby so that he also can experience a realistic completion of this part of his life.

58. **D.** All of the factors mentioned will contribute to the high-risk category of this teenager.

59. **C.** The lack of prenatal care that many unmarried teenagers receive accounts for much of the

high rate of prematurity and infant mortality found in their offspring.

60. **D.** All of the complications mentioned can be found in the adolescent girl during pregnancy.

61. **B.** The teenage girl needs about 1.3 g of calcium to meet her own body needs. The increased need for calcium during pregnancy raises her calcium requirement to 1.7 g daily.

62. **A.** The recommended intake of milk during the adolescent period is one quart; therefore, an additional glass of milk should equal the necessary milk intake.

63. **D.** The emotional stress caused by pregnancy, added to the already stressful period of adolescence, may contribute to the low level of essential nutrients.

64. **D.** The adolescent girl may have an erratic diet simply because she is in that stage of her development. She may come from a low socioeconomic home where high-quality food is simply not available. As a result of the stress of pregnancy, she may overeat, or, as more commonly happens, she may starve herself as a punishment for the act itself.

65. **C.** The unmarried mother may have many problems at this time. Although the nurse may not be equipped to handle some of these problems, she can be most helpful by just spending time with the girl and by listening to what is being said.

66. **C.** The unwed mother may expect the labor and delivery experience to be one in which she will be punished for her wrongdoings. Therefore, extra time should be taken to make sure that she is made as comfortable as possible.

67. **D.** The unwed mother who gives birth to an abnormal child will have great feelings of guilt, assuming that this is her punishment for conceiving the child out of wedlock.

68. **C.** The Child Welfare League of America is the agency that establishes the standards for adoptive practices.

69. **C.** It is important for the girl to be an active participant in the final parts of this childbearing experience. Only in this way can she experience a sense of completion in the total experience of childbearing.

70. **D.** About 10% of all American families are headed by a woman.

71. **D.** In 1970 approximately 43% of all women held full-time positions outside the home.

72. **C.** With the change in the American family, more women are able to raise children in the single-parent family without the severe rejection from society that has been the case.

73. **A.** It is felt that the sexually active teenager has not yet been reached with effective contraception and that the girls who are likely to conceive should have complete access to contraceptive education and methods.

74. **B.** The hormones in the contraceptive pills may lead to premature closure of the epiphysis.

75. **D.** All of the factors mentioned are considered to be problems in teenage family planning programs.

76. **C.** The ideal age for reproduction appears to be between the ages of 25 and 30.

77. **B.** The first birth control clinic in the United States was opened in 1916 by Margaret Sanger in a Brooklyn slum.

78. **A.** Margaret Sanger formed the Planned Parenthood Federation of America, Inc., in 1942.

79. **C.** Planned Parenthood—World Population was established in 1960 when Planned Parenthood Federation of America, Inc. and the International Planned Parenthood Federation merged into one organization.

80. **D.** The Margaret Sanger Research Bureau was established in 1923. This organization was created for the purpose of providing research in the field of infertility, contraception, and marriage counseling.

81. **D.** The diaphragm was first introduced in the 1800s.

82. **B.** About 5% of women in planned parenthood clinics choose the diaphragm as a contraceptive method.

83. **B.** The failure rate for women who use the diaphragm *correctly* is about three pregnancies per year. In actual use and effectiveness, however, there may be ten to fifteen pregnancies per 100 women per year.

84. **D.** The diaphragm should be left in place for at least six hours after coitus.

85. **C.** Women object to the insertion, checking the position, and removal of the diaphragm.

86. **B.** Although the diaphragm does act as a mechanical barrier against the entry of the sperm into the cervix, its primary function is to hold the spermicidal jelly or cream.

87. **C.** In 1960 the first hormonal contraceptives were introduced in the United States.

88. **B.** The sequential type of birth control pill first suppressed the follicle-stimulating hormone and then both the follicle-stimulating and luteinizing hormones.

89. **D.** There are more than 30 different oral contraceptives available in the United States.

90. **C.** About 50% of women ovulate and menstruate in their first postpill cycle.

91. **D.** All of the symptoms mentioned should be reported to the doctor.

92. **B.** Estrogen is a gastrointestinal irritant.

93. **C.** The physician who inserts the IUD during the last few days of the menstrual cycle can be assured that there is not a pre-existing pregnancy. Also, the slight bleeding that may occur as a result of the insertion is not as alarming to the patient because it is taken as part of the menstrual period.

94. **D.** The symptoms mentioned are considered to be the side effects of oral contraceptives.

95. **B.** The failure rate for women who retain the IUD is about 2% during the first year. However, this rate declines in later years.

96. **D.** However, many theories have been advanced regarding the action of the intra-uterine contraceptive devices, such as those stated in A, B, and C.

97. **C.** The nylon tab attached to the end of the IUD that extends from the vaginal canal is called the cervical appendage.

98. **C.** The rhythm method is based on determining the expected date of ovulation and then refraining from sexual intercourse during those days when conception could occur.

99. **A.** The woman's temperature is at its lowest during the secretory phase of the menstrual cycle. At the time of ovulation, the woman's temperature rises suddenly and sharply. The ovum has a life of 24 hours or less.

100. **D.** The rhythm method is not a satisfactory method for women who have irregular menses, and it may fail because of early, unexpected ovulation or delayed ovulation.

101. **B.** The rhythm method is also referred to as periodic continence, temporary abstinence, or safe period.

102. **C.** In using this method, the man withdraws his penis from the vagina immediately before ejaculation.

103. **D.** Despite the self-control factor on the part of the husband and the anxiety that can be produced in the woman, there is a small amount of semen in the pre-ejaculatory secretion.

104. **A.** The condom was introduced primarily as a defense against veneral disease.

105. **D.** The condom is known by all the names listed.

106. **C.** The condom has an accidental pregnancy rate of about 3%.

107. **D.** Douching should be postponed for at least six hours after coitus.

108. **C.** Spermicidal preparations should be inserted within one hour before coitus.

109. **B.** Vaginal suppositories should be inserted about 10 minutes before coitus to allow them to melt.

110. **A.** Foaming tablets should be inserted about five minutes before coitus.

111. **A.** The oral contraceptives are being selected by about 75% of patients being seen in the planned parenthood clinics.

112. **C.** The spermatozoa enter the uterus within 90 seconds following the depositing of the semen at the cervical os, and the majority of spermatozoa are contained in the first few drops of semen. Therefore, postcoital douching is of little benefit in flushing the semen out of the vagina before they can enter the uterus.

113. **A.** The diaphragm should not be left in place during the entire menstrual cycle.

114. **B.** The oral hormones act by inhibiting ovulation, and if taken correctly provide a high degree of effectiveness.

115. **C.** During ovulation there is an increase in the amount of mucus secreted by the cervical glands, with its resultant escape from the vaginal canal.

116. **B.** The Sims-Huhner test is a postcoital examination of cervical mucus. It is done at the time of ovulation and from one to twelve hours after coitus.

117. **B.** Vasectomy takes 20 to 30 minutes in the doctors' office or in an out-patient department.

118. **C.** Male sterilization is considered to be reversible in about 20 to 40% of cases.

119. **C.** The semen should be examined after about 10 ejaculations or after about 8 weeks to insure that it is sperm-free.

120. **B.** Connecticut in 1821 passed a law that made abortion a criminal offense.

121. **B.** Aleck Bourne in 1938 performed an abortion on a 14-year-old girl who had been raped by soldiers. Then he notified the police. His acquittal provided the first liberalized guidelines for practicing physicians.

122. **A.** Age distribution of women shows that 59.4% of abortions were obtained by women between the ages of 16 and 24.

123. **B.** The data here show that 47.1% of legal abortions were done between the ninth and twelfth week of gestation.

124. **D.** During this time the fallopian tubes are more readily accessible.

125. **B.** Although all are involved in doing laparoscopic tubal sterilization, the Falope ring and spring-loaded clip avoid the thermal hazard associated with cautery.

126. **B.** The hazard associated with laparoscopic sterilization is carbon dioxide embolism.

127. **D.** In January, 1973, the United States Supreme Court handed the mentioned degree and also indicated that decisions to seek abortions during the second and third trimester are subject to regulations and laws of the individual states.

128. **C.** This procedure is called menstrual extraction, and the abortion is caused by evacuating the uterus immediately after the woman misses a period.

129. **A.** It has been shown by several investigators that using dilatation and curettage as a method of abortion increases the number of fetal erythrocytes in the mother's blood. Therefore, all Rh negative patients should be given RhoGAM following the procedure to eliminate the possibility of Rh sensitization.

130. **B.** Prostaglandin is the name given to the fatty acid extract found in human seminal fluid.

131. **A.** Ulf Svante von Euler was the 1970 Nobel Laureate who noted that this component was a fatty acid extract secreted by the seminal vessel and named it prostaglandin.

132. **A.** Dr. Sultan M. Karim of Uganda discovered that a high concentration of two of the prostaglandins circulate through the venous blood of women during labor.

133. **B.** The symptoms mentioned are the result of excessive progesterone in the body.

134. **B.** The side effects of intravenous prostaglandins include gastrointestinal difficulties (nausea, vomiting, and diarrhea) and erythema overlying the vein used for infusion.

135. **B.** The largest number of abortions were obtained by women between the ages of 15 and 24 in the year 1973.

136. **B.** D and E was used in 40.8% of all abortions, and the D and C was used in 34.8% of all cases.

137. **C.** Following a saline amnioinfusion, labor usually starts within 12 to 36 hours.

138. **C.** In a saline amnioinfusion, fetal death can occur within an hour.

139. **B.** About 150 to 200 mL of fluid is removed from the uterus, and an equal amount of a 20% hypertonic saline solution is injected back into the uterus.

140. **D.** Saline infusion causes diffuse intravascular coagulation and can cause significant bleeding within 24 hours of the procedure, with fever and bacteremia.

141. **B.** Doctors recommend that a D and C be performed on primigravidas before the tenth week of gestation.

142. **C.** Saline amnioinfusion is used during the second trimester after the fourteenth week.

143. **C.** There is a predicted complication rate of about 5% for women having abortions early in pregnancy.

144. **D.** All of the complications mentioned can occur as a result of abortions.

145. **C.** There is a predicted complication rate of about 20% for women having abortions late in pregnancy.

146. **D.** Dr. Grantly Dick Read published the book *Natural Childbirth* in 1933.

147. **B.** This society, also known as ASPO, was organized in 1960 and is composed of three divisions: physicians, teachers, and parents.

148. **C.** Read method principles were first instituted in 1945 under the direction of Dr. Herbert Thomas.

149. **C.** The International Childbirth Education Association was founded in 1960.

150. **B.** He was a London obstetrician and responsible for the original natural childbirth movement in London.

151. **C.** Preparation, according to this school of thought, deals with training in conditioned responses to the uterine contractions.

152. **C.** Marjorie Karmel's book *Thank you, Dr. Lamaze* was published in the early 1950s.

153. **B.** Dr. Clement Yahia introduced this method during the year 1960.

154. **A.** The two Russian doctors, Nicolaiev and Velvovskiy were the first to advocate this method of childbirth.

155. **C.** Psychoprophylaxis started in Russia in 1949.

156. **C.** Ivan Pavlov proved this theory by ringing a bell while placing food before a dog. The dog became conditioned to salivate simply by hearing the bell, but without receiving the food. Dr. Lamaze utilized this theory of learned reaction to stimuli through training in developing his method of natural childbirth.

157. **D.** Ideally, the Lamaze method should be taught during the last six weeks of pregnancy. If taught too early, there may be a loss of motivation on the part of the woman, and if taught too late, there may not be enough time to cover all of the content.

158. **B.** The goal of the Lamaze method is to prepare the woman to control the amount of discomfort that results from the labor and delivery process.

159. **B.** Motherliness usually starts during the earliest months with maternal-infant interaction (maternal claiming process).

160. **B.** The exercises used to prepare the mother emphasize an approach based on the principles of relaxation and are conducted with the total program.

161. **D.** All of the factors mentioned are important when attempting to do health teaching in the group setting.

162. **C.** In the group setting, every member of the group has expertise about some aspects. Therefore, the group leader should function only as the resource person, adding information where no one else can contribute it.

163. **C.** In this type of setting, group members contribute the topics for discussion, and the leader simply keeps the discussion going and raises points to help the group members discuss the chosen topic more completely.

164. **C.** Education for both expectant parents should be broadly based and include issues beyond the pregnancy cycle if these bear a relationship to the topic.

165. **B.** The LaLeche League was organized by six mothers in Franklin Park, Illinois, in 1956.

166. **B.** Support and encouragement of women who are breast feeding is one of the main goals of the LaLeche League.

167. **C.** Abdominal breathing is done during labor to lift up the abdominal wall from the uterus so there is less discomfort during a contraction.

168. **B.** The purpose of tailor sitting during pregnancy is that of stretching the thighs and pelvic floor muscles.

169. **B.** Cornelian Corner, organized in 1942 in Detroit, Michigan, represented the first organized effort to free infant care from the rigid standards that had prevailed for the past 20 years. This group stressed the need for rooming-in.

170. **B.** This type of setting provides the mother with the advantages of hospital care in a home-like environment. The program focuses on a family-centered approach where both mother and father can learn about the new child and how to provide care to him.

171. **A.** *The Prospective Mother* was written by Dr. Josiah Morris Stemons in 1912 and emphasized the hygiene of pregnancy.

172. **B.** *Prenatal Care* was first published in 1913 and *Infant Care* in 1914 by the Children's Bureau.

173. **C.** The purposes of exercises are to promote comfort during pregnancy, to facilitate childbirth, and to aid in strengthening muscles during the puerperium.

174. **A.** The woman's concerns during this time are with herself and with the changes that are taking place within her body.

175. **B.** During the second trimester the woman turns her attention toward the life within her.

176. **C.** The woman now waits expectantly for labor and needs to know about the labor and delivery process.

177. **C.** With this exercise there is the possible danger of a fatal air embolism when air has entered the vagina.

178. **B.** On or about the third day, the mother has moved out of the "taking-in" phase and is ready to start taking hold. Essentially she is physically and psychologically ready to start learning about her new role and its responsibilities.

179. **C.** The first trained nurse-midwife was used in the Frontier Nursing Service.

180. **B.** The Maternity Center Association was founded in New York in 1918.

181. **D.** The woman's concept of the mother role is based on all of the factors mentioned.

182. **D.** The American College of Nurse-Midwifery was established in 1955.

183. **B.** The founder of the Frontier Nursing Service was Mary Breckinridge.

184. **C.** The Maternity Center Association established the first school of nurse-midwifery in 1932. The Lobenstine Midwifery Clinic was established at this time to provide a field service for the school.

185. **D.** The Frontier Graduate School of Midwifery started its program in 1939.

186. **C.** There are approximately 15 nurse-midwifery programs in the United States.

187. **C.** The American College of Nurse-Midwifery recognizes that nurse-midwives function not as independent practitioners but as health workers within the framework of a medically directed health service in which the physician is ultimately responsible for each patient's care.

188. **B.** The American College of Nurse-Midwifery became a member of the International Confederation of Midwives in 1957.

189. **D.** All of the functions mentioned are inherent in the role of the nurse-midwife.

190. **C.** Carolyn Van Blarcom was the first nurse in the United States to take out a midwifery license and register as a nurse-midwife.

191. **A.** The purpose of this book on midwifery was to give advice on how the life of the child could be saved until he was baptized.

192. **B.** The midwife is referred to in Exodus 1:16-20.

193. **B.** Bellevue Hospital is given credit for being the first hospital in the United States to give instructions in midwifery.

194. **B.** Dr. Attwood was from New York and his name was recorded in 1745.

195. **C.** Hendrik van Deventer of Holland, "father of modern midwifery," showed much determination in bringing about male participation in midwifery.

196. **C.** At this time there is a definite lack of the services, equipment, and techniques necessary for a safe delivery within the home. For this reason, the majority of women are encouraged to have their deliveries within the hospital.

197. **B.** In 1935 only about 37% of all deliveries were done within the hospital.

198. **C.** About 94% of nonwhite deliveries are being conducted in the hospital, whereas almost 100% of white deliveries are being done in the hospital.

199. **B.** Ambrose Pare of Paris was a great medical leader of the sixteenth century. He described the podalic version and made this procedure more practicable.

200. **A.** Francois Mauriceau of France was a leader in obstetrics during the seventeenth century. He dispensed with the use of the obstetrical chair for delivery and started using the bed instead.

201. **C.** Hendrik van Deventer of Holland also wrote a book that gave the first accurate description of the pelvis and how pelvic deformities complicated labor.

202. **D.** William Smellie of London also introduced the still-locked forceps.

203. **C.** The United Nations International Children's Emergency Fund is concerned with the health and welfare of children and mothers.

204. **A.** The World Health Organization is interested in the attainment of the highest possible level of health throughout the world.

205. **B.** The Children's Bureau provides leadership in instituting and coordinating child and parent programs.

206. **D.** The International Social Service provides assistance to the homeless child.

207. **C.** Irwin Chabon wrote *Awake and Aware* in 1966.

208. **D.** Helen Heardman, an English physiotherapist, wrote *A Way to Natural Childbirth*. In this book she describes the exercise, breathing, and relaxation techniques taught in natural childbirth classes.

209. **A.** *Revelation of Childbirth* was published in England in 1944 by Dr. Grantly Dick Read. This same book was published in the United States under the title of *Childbirth Without Fear*.

210. **B.** Alene Auerbach, while associated with the Child Study Association of America, wrote *Parents Learn Through Discussion*. Ms. Auerbach is a recognized leader in the parent education movement.

211. **D.** The Mauriceau's maneuver is used when the physician is delivering a child that is in the breech position.

212. **A.** The Scanzoni maneuver is used to rotate the head presenting in an occiput posterior position to an occiput anterior position.

213. **C.** The Ritgen's maneuver is used to control the delivery of the head in an occiput anterior position.

214. **B.** The Leopold's maneuver is used to determine the presentation and position of the baby by abdominal palpation.

CHAPTER 2

Anatomy and Physiology of the Female and Male Reproductive Systems

The ability of individuals to produce a child is often related to the state of their own body functioning.

Included in this chapter are questions on the internal and external organs of reproduction and the part played by the body hormones. Presented here are various points pertaining to the female pelvis and to the baby who must pass through this structure during the birth process.

It is important, therefore, to understand the basis of female and male anatomy and physiology as related to childbirth.

Directions: Each of the questions or incomplete statements below is followed by four suggested answers or completions. Select the BEST answer in each case.

1. Collectively, the external genitalia of women are most commonly called the
   A. pudendum
   B. perineum
   C. vulva
   D. none of the above   (8:3)

2. The external genitalia of women include
   A. all externally visible organs
   B. all externally visible organs situated in the perineal area
   C. all externally visible organs extending from the area over the symphysis pubis to the base of the perineal body
   D. none of the above   (8:3)

3. The mons veneris can best be described by which of the following statements?
   A. firm pad of adipose and connective tissue that lies over the symphysis pubis and adjoining pubic bones
   B. heavy ridges of adipose and connective tissue that forms lateral boundaries of the vulva

   C. small cylindrical body composed of erectile tissue located at the upper aspect of the vulva
   D. none of the above   (8:3)

4. The vestibule can best be described as
   A. the triangular area formed by the labia minora
   B. the triangular area formed by the labia majora
   C. the triangular area visible between the clitoris and the anus
   D. none of the above   (8:5)

5. The urinary meatus can best be located in the woman
   A. at the point where the labia minora join anteriorly
   B. at the apex of the triangle when the labia minora are spread apart
   C. in the midline of the vestibule below the clitoris and above the vaginal orifice
   D. none of the above   (8:5)

6. The vaginal orifice can best be located in the woman by which of the following descriptions?
   A. midline of the vestibule
   B. upper portion of the vestibule

C. lower portion of the vestibule
D. none of the above (8:5)

7. The labia minora can best be described by which of the following statements?

A. longitudinal folds of adipose tissue that extend posteriorly to form the beginning of the perineum
B. longitudinal folds of cutaneous tissue that extend from the clitoris downward and backward on either side of the vaginal orifice
C. almond-shaped area that extends backward from the clitoris to the fourchette
D. none of the above (8:4)

8. Which of the following structures tends to remain somewhat relaxed following childbirth?

A. labia minora
B. labia majora
C. vestibule
D. urinary meatus (8:4)

9. The hood-like covering over the clitoris is termed the

A. hymen
B. fourchette
C. prepuce
D. frenulum (8:4)

10. Which one of the following glands is found in the vagina?

A. Skene's glands
B. apocrine glands
C. Bartholin's glands
D. none of the above (8:13)

11. Which of the following are considered to be functions of the Bartholin's glands?

1. provide smegma within folds of the labia
2. provide acidic reaction in the vagina
3. provide lubrication to vaginal orifice and canal
4. provide moisture to inner surfaces of the labia

A. 1, 2, 3
B. 3, 4
C. 1, 3, 4
D. all of the above (8:6)

12. The Skene's glands in women are analogous to what gland in men?

A. Cowper's glands
B. prostate gland

C. Bartholin's glands
D. none of the above (2:53)

13. The vestibular bulb is

A. the anterior portion of the vestibule
B. a collection of veins located on either side of the vagina beneath the mucous membranes
C. the posterior portion of the vestibule
D. the depressed space between the vaginal opening and the fourchette (2:54)

14. The fornix is located

A. between the uterus and the bladder
B. between the cervix and the vaginal wall
C. between the uterus and fallopian tubes
D. none of the above (8:14)

15. Which one of the following female organs is analogous to the male penis?

A. fallopian tube
B. uterus
C. clitoris
D. ovary (4:75)

16. The perineal body is located

A. between the lower aspect of the symphysis pubis and the rectum
B. between the uppermost aspect of the symphysis pubis and the rectum
C. between the vagina and the rectum
D. within the vestibule (8:7)

17. The pelvic diaphragm is located

A. between the bladder and the uterus
B. in the uppermost part of the pelvic cavity
C. in the lowermost part of the pelvic cavity
D. between the uterus and the rectum (8:6)

18. The purpose of the pelvic diaphragm is

A. to serve as a support for abdominal organs
B. to serve as a support for pelvic organs
C. to assist in the constriction of vagina, rectum, and anus
D. all of the above (8:6)

19. The pelvic diaphragm is composed of which of the following muscles?

A. coccygeus muscles and transverse perinei
B. levator ani and coccygeus muscles

C. transverse perinei and sphincter vaginae

D. levator ani and sphincter vaginae (8:6)

20. The term perineum is used in obstetrics when speaking about which of the following?

A. the area between the fourchette and anus

B. the area between the pubic arch and the anus

C. the area between the symphysis pubis and the vestibule

D. none of these (6:4)

21. Which of the following muscles are considered to be part of the perineum?

1. coccygeus muscles
2. bulbocavernosus
3. transverse perineal muscles
4. levator ani
5. uterosacral ligament

A. 1

B. 2, 3

C. 1, 2, 3, 4

D. all of these (8:7)

22. In the woman who has never been pregnant, which of the following observations would be considered normal?

A. carunculae myrtiformes

B. external os of cervix, small round opening

C. laceration of perineal tissues

D. gaping labia majora (8:6,11,386)

23. The normal pH value of the cervical mucus at the time of ovulation is

A. about 4

B. between 5 and 6

C. close to 7.5

D. none of these (8:38)

24. The diameter of the cervix is approximately

A. 0.25 in.

B. 0.50 in.

C. 0.75 in.

D. 1 in. (8:11)

25. The cervix is approximately how long?

A. 0.5 to 1 cm

B. 1 to 1.5 cm

C. 2 to 2.5 cm

D. 2.5 to 3 cm (8:11)

26. The fossa navicularis is located

A. at the opening of the vagina

B. between the fourchette and vaginal orifice

C. in the upper part of the vestibule

D. in none of the above places (6:4)

27. The cul-de-sac of Douglas is located

A. in the upper aspect of the uterus

B. in the lower aspect of the uterus

C. between the lower part of the uterus and the rectum

D. between the lower part of the uterus and the bladder (6:5)

28. Anatomically, what is the name given to the area that lies externally between the thighs and extends from the pubic area to the coccyx?

A. pelvic diaphragm

B. perineum

C. perineal body

D. none of the above (8:7)

29. The normal pH value of the vaginal secretions during the childbearing years is usually

A. about 3

B. between 4.0 and 5.0

C. between 5.5 and 6.5

D. above 6.5 (8:13)

30. Colporrhaphy is

A. observation of the vagina during a routine examination

B. an operation during which the vagina is sutured

C. visual inspection of the Douglas' cul-de-sac

D. none of the above (4:617)

31. The breasts are considered to be

A. internal organs of reproduction

B. external organs of reproduction

C. accessory organs of reproduction

D. not part of the glands of reproduction (2:59)

32. Approximately how many lobes are there in each breast?

A. 5 to 10

B. 10 to 15

C. 15 to 20

D. 20 to 25 (2:59)

33. Which of the following open into the tip of the nipple?

A. tubercles of Montgomery

B. lactiferous ducts

C.   lactiferous sinus
D.   aerolar glands   (2:59)

34. Which of the following vessels does *not* supply blood to the breast?

A.   thoracic branches of the axillary arteries
B.   pudendal artery
C.   intercostal arteries
D.   internal thoracic arteries   (2:59)

35. Which of the following provide the major source of blood to the perineum?

A.   inferior hemorrhoidal artery
B.   pudendal artery
C.   both A and B
D.   neither A nor B   (6:5)

36. Nerve innervation to the breasts comes from the

1. third thoracic nerve
2. fourth thoracic nerve
3. fifth thoracic nerve
4. sixth thoracic nerve
5. supraclavicular nerves

A.   1, 2, 3, 4
B.   5
C.   2, 3, 4, 5
D.   all of these   (6:8)

37. In the adult woman the breasts weigh approximately how much?

A.   50 to 100 g
B.   100 to 200 g
C.   200 to 250 g
D.   200 to 300 g   (6:8)

38. The circular area in the center of the breast is called the

A.   papilla
B.   areola
C.   chloasma
D.   striae gravidarium   (6:8)

39. Another name for the nipple is

A.   mammary gland
B.   mammary papilla
C.   Montgomery's tubercle
D.   none of these   (6:8)

40. The nipple is primarily composed of

A.   cutaneous tissue
B.   fat tissue
C.   fibromuscular tissue
D.   all of the above   (6:8)

41. The structure most directly involved in the production of milk is the

A.   papillae
B.   glands of Montgomery
C.   acini or alveoli
D.   lactiferous ducts   (4:82)

42. Which of the following organs is *not* considered to be an internal organ of reproduction?

A.   uterus
B.   fallopian tubes
C.   ovaries
D.   clitoris   (5:16)

43. The uterus functions as the organ that

A.   produces the ovum
B.   transports the ovum
C.   houses the ovum
D.   none of the above   (8:9)

44. The layers of the muscular uterus are termed

A.   ectoderm, mesoderm, endoderm
B.   endometrium, myometrium, perimetrium
C.   basalis, capsularis, vera
D.   none of the above   (5:18)

45. The uterus is supplied with blood by the

A.   abdominal aorta and uterine arteries
B.   internal iliac and ovarian arteries
C.   ovarian and uterine arteries
D.   internal iliac and uterine arteries   (5:19)

46. The upper, rounded portion of the uterus between the insertion of the fallopian tubes is called the

A.   fundus
B.   corpus
C.   isthmus
D.   cornua   (5:19)

47. The junction between the body of the uterus and the cervix is called the

A.   Bandl's ring
B.   fornix
C.   isthmus
D.   none of the above   (8:9−10)

48. The muscular tissue of the uterus is

A.   primarily striated
B.   primarily nonstriated
C.   entirely striated
D.   entirely nonstriated   (5:19)

49. The nerve supply to the uterus is derived primarily from the
    A. cerebrospinal system
    B. sympathetic system
    C. parasympathetic system
    D. none of the above   (4:79)

50. The *chief* support for the uterus is provided by the
    A. transverse broad ligament
    B. cardinal ligaments
    C. round ligaments
    D. uterosacral ligaments   (6:6)

51. Which of the following statements best describes the function of the uterosacral ligaments?
    A. assist in keeping the uterus from prolapsing by providing support from below
    B. assist in keeping the uterus in its normal position by exerting traction on the cervix
    C. both A and B
    D. neither A nor B   (8:12)

52. Which one of the following is *not* considered to be a function of the ovaries?
    A. development of the ova
    B. expulsion of the ova
    C. provision of internal secretions
    D. none of the above   (4:77)

53. Which of the following are considered to be the function(s) of the ovary?
    A. they secrete hormones necessary for the cycle changes in the endometrium
    B. they produce secondary oocytes
    C. they release the oocytes
    D. all of the above   (6:6)

54. The inner layer of the ovary is called the
    A. cortex
    B. medulla
    C. stroma
    D. cytoplasm   (6:6)

55. The ovaries are suspended by folds of peritoneum called
    A. mesosalpinx
    B. mesovarium
    C. frenulum
    D. rugae   (6:6)

56. What is the name of the portion of the fallopian tube that lies very near to the ovary and transports the ovum to its point of fertilization?
    A. fimbriae
    B. fimbria ovarica
    C. infundibulum
    D. none of the above   (8:15)

57. The distal opening of the fallopian tube is called the
    A. interstitial portion
    B. isthmus
    C. ampulla
    D. infundibulum   (8:14)

58. Each fallopian tube is approximately how long?
    A. 4 to 6 in.
    B. 7 to 14 in.
    C. 10 to 16 in.
    D. 12 to 20 in.   (2:54)

59. The fallopian tubes are lined with
    A. serous membrane
    B. circular fibers
    C. mucous membrane
    D. longitudinal fibers   (4:78)

60. The fallopian tubes possess a nerve supply from the
    A. sympathetic nervous system
    B. cerebrospinal system
    C. parasympathetic system
    D. all of the above   (4:78−80)

61. The ovum is transported from the ovary to the uterus by
    A. the cilia, which create a current in the capillary layer of fluid lying between the various pelvic organs
    B. the musculature within the tubes, which undergoes rhythmic contractions
    C. the movement of the cilia within the tube, which provides a one-way action
    D. all of the above   (4:78)

62. Which one of the following male organs is analogous to the ovary in the woman?
    A. prostate gland
    B. testes
    C. bulbourethral glands
    D. epididymis   (8:18)

63. Which one of the following is *not* part of the canal system which carries the sperm to the external world?
    A. testes
    B. epididymis

C. vas deferens
D. urethra   (2:61)

64. Which of the following structures of the male reproductive system is responsible for sperm transportation from the testes to the urethra?

A. testicle
B. vas deferens
C. prostate gland
D. seminiferous vesicle   (8:22)

65. The internal organs of the male reproductive system are

A. scrotum, penis
B. scrotum, testes, penis
C. testes, canal system, accessory structures
D. testes, canal system   (4:84)

66. Which of the following is *not* considered to be an accessory structure in the male reproductive system?

A. seminal vesicles
B. vas deferens
C. prostate gland
D. Cowper's gland   (2:61)

67. The tubules within the testes are called

A. tubercles of Montgomery
B. seminiferous tubules
C. rete testis
D. none of the above   (8:18)

68. The testes descend into the scrotum at about

A. the fourth month of fetal life
B. the seventh or eighth month of fetal life
C. the first month of extrauterine life
D. puberty   (8:18)

69. The seminiferous tubules are about how long?

A. 3 to 6 in.
B. 6 to 12 in.
C. 1 to 3 ft.
D. 2 to 4 ft.   (8:19)

70. The purpose of the germinal epithelium in the seminiferous tubules is to

A. provide secretions that are mixed with the germ cells
B. produce immature germ cells
C. nourish and maintain germ cells
D. none of the above   (8:19)

71. The seminiferous tubules come together and form a single coiled tube called the

A. rete testis
B. epididymis
C. vas deferens
D. urethra   (2:61)

72. The blood supply to the testes is derived from

A. internal spermatic arteries
B. inferior hemorrhoidal
C. uterovaginal plexus
D. pudendal arteries   (4:84)

73. The vas deferentia are about how long?

A. 6 in.
B. 12 in.
C. 18 in.
D. 24 in.   (8:22)

74. The pH of semen varies from

A. 6.5 to 7
B. 7.35 to 7.50
C. 7.60 to 7.75
D. none of the above   (8:24)

75. The enlargement at the end of the penis is called the

A. prepuce
B. foreskin
C. glans penis
D. none of the above   (8:24)

76. Why is the pelvis considered important from an obstetrical viewpoint?

A. it is the cavity that contains the generative organs
B. it is the basin-shaped cavity formed by the hip bones and the end of the backbone
C. it is the canal through which the baby must pass during birth
D. A and C   (4:65)

77. The pelvis is made up of four united bones. Which of the following is *not* one of these bones?

A. two hip bones
B. symphysis pubis
C. sacrum
D. coccyx   (4:65−6)

78. The two hip bones are joined together anteriorly by the

A. symphysis pubis
B. sacroiliac joints
C. sacrococcygeal joint
D. thick bones   (8:243)

79. Which one of the following bones is mova-
   ble, thus providing more space for passage
   of the baby at the time of birth?

   A. sacrum
   B. coccyx
   C. ilium
   D. ischium (8:245)

80. Which part of the pelvis is used as an important landmark during internal pelvic
   measurements?

   A. iliac crests
   B. coccyx
   C. sacral promontory
   D. hip bones (4:66)

81. During the latter months of pregnancy the
   woman may suffer from backaches and leg
   aches. This is due to

   A. growing fetus in the uterus
   B. excessive weight gain
   C. engagement of the baby in the pelvis
   D. increased mobility of the articulations
      of the pelvis (8:245)

82. The pelvis consists of two parts: the true
   pelvis and the false pelvis. The false pelvis is
   important because

   A. it supports the uterus and plays a part
      in the actual birth of the baby
   B. it supports the uterus and directs the
      fetus into the true pelvis at the proper
      time
   C. it supports the uterus and is important
      in external pelvimetry
   D. B and C (4:67–8)

83. The true pelvis consists of three parts.
   Which one of the following is *not* considered
   to be a part of the true pelvis?

   A. inlet
   B. cavity
   C. ilium
   D. outlet (4:68)

84. The pelvic inlet can best be described by
   which of the following statements?

   A. roughly heart-shaped, widest from
      back to front and narrowest from side
      to side
   B. roughly heart-shaped, widest from side
      to side and narrowest from back to
      front
   C. roughly oval-shaped, equal distance
      from side to side and back to front

   D. roughly oval-shaped, widest from side
      to side and narrowest from back to
      front (4:68)

85. The pelvic cavity is situated between the
   inlet and the outlet. Its shape can best be
   described as

   A. cylindrical, with upper parts curved
      and lower portion straight
   B. cylindrical, with upper parts straight
      and lower portion curved
   C. cylindrical, with both upper and lower
      parts straight
   D. cylindrical, with both upper and lower
      parts curved (2:57)

86. The pelvic outlet can best be described as

   A. a space bounded in front by the
      symphysis pubis, at the sides by the is-
      chial tuberosities, and behind by the
      coccyx and greater sacrosciatic liga-
      ments
   B. a space bounded in front by the
      symphysis pubis, at the back by the
      sacral promontory, and at the sides by
      the hip bones
   C. a space bounded in front by the
      symphysis pubis, at the sides and back
      of the superior strait
   D. none of the above (4:68)

87. The true and false pelvis are separated by an
   imaginary line termed

   A. linea alba
   B. linea terminalis
   C. linea nigra
   D. none of the above (2:57)

88. Complete maturing of the pelvis takes place
   during which of the following age spans?

   A. 8 to 12
   B. 12 to 16
   C. 16 to 20
   D. 20 to 25 (4:69)

89. Which of the following statements describes
   the gynecoid or female pelvis?

   A. pelvic inlet is deep in hind- and fore-
      pelvis, increased in the anteroposterior
      diameter; sacrosciatic notch is broad
      and shallow
   B. pelvic inlet is a transverse oval, well
      curved but decreases in the anteropos-
      terior diameter; sacrosciatic notch is
      curved and small
   C. pelvic inlet is well rounded in hind- and
      fore-pelvic; sacrosciatic notch is

curved, moderate in width and depth

D. pelvic inlet is wedge-shaped, with shallow hind-pelvis and pointed fore-pelvis; sacrosciatic notch is narrow and deeply pointed (4:70)

90. Why is it important to obtain an accurate determination of the pelvic measurements during pregnancy?

A. although the body stature of a woman may appear to be within normal limits, the pelvis may not be within normal limits

B. slight irregularities in the structure of the pelvis may delay the progress of labor

C. marked deformity may prohibit the possibility of a vaginal delivery

D. all of the above (4:71)

91. Which of the following is considered to be the most accurate way to determine the pelvic measurements?

A. external measurements
B. internal measurements
C. x-ray pelvimetry
D. combination of A and B (2:58−9)

92. External measurements are accomplished with a pelvimeter and a Thomas retractor while the mother is lying flat on the examining table. Which of the following is considered to be the most important external measurement?

A. intercrestal diameter
B. intertrochanteric diameter
C. external conjugate diameter
D. bi-ischial (or intertuberous) diameter (5:30−1)

93. Internal measurements are accomplished by a palpation of the doctor's fingers while the mother is in lithotomy position with her feet supported in stirrups. Which of the following is the most important internal measurement?

A. diagonal conjugate
B. ischial spines diameter
C. degree of pubic arch
D. none of the above (4:71−2)

94. Which of the following numbers best indicates the expected diameter of the diagonal conjugate?

A. 11.0 cm
B. 12.5 cm

C. 25 cm
D. 28 cm (4:72)

95. Why is the length of the true conjugate (or conjugate vera) considered to be of importance in obstetrics?

A. it is the smallest diameter of the inlet through which the baby's head must pass

B. it is the smallest diameter of the outlet through which the baby's head must pass

C. it is the widest diameter of the outlet through which the baby's head must pass

D. it is the widest diameter of the inlet through which the baby's head must pass (4:72)

96. The intertuberous diameter measurement is taken by determining the distance between the

A. lateral edges of the iliac crests
B. external aspects of the trochanters of the femurs
C. two ischial spines
D. two ischial tuberosities (4:73)

97. The anteroposterior diameter of the outlet extends from the

A. middle of the lower margin of the symphysis pubis to the tip of the sacrum

B. lower margin of the symphysis pubis through the area between the ischial spines to the sacrum

C. upper margins of the pubic bones to the sacral promontory

D. none of these (8:249

98. The posterior sagittal diameter is the distance

A. from the top of the symphysis pubis to the sacral promontory

B. from the midpoint of an imaginary line between the ischial tuberosities to the tip of the sacrum

C. between the anterior aspect of one ilium to the other ilium

D. none of these (8:250)

99. The ischial tuberosities are found on the lower end of the

A. ilium
B. ischium
C. pubis
D. sacrum (8:244)

100. Which of the following sets of landmarks is used to determine the shortest diameter of the pelvic cavity?
    A. anterior-superior iliac spines
    B. ischial tuberosities
    C. ischial spines
    D. none of the above   (8:244)

101. In the normal standing position, the plane of the pelvic brim is
    A. exactly horizontal
    B. tilted forward
    C. tilted backward
    D. exactly vertical   (8:245)

102. The pubic arch is the portion of the
    A. bone above the symphysis pubis
    B. true pelvis extending from one ischial tuberosity to the other
    C. bony pelvis through which the baby passes
    D. true pelvis above the ischial tuberosity   (5:32)

103. The sacrum is joined to the two hip bones by the
    A. symphysis pubis
    B. sacroiliac joints
    C. sacral promontory
    D. linea terminales   (8:245)

104. The transverse diameter is the
    A. smallest diameter of the inlet
    B. greatest width of the inlet
    C. greatest width of the pelvic cavity
    D. smallest width of the pelvic cavity   (8:247)

105. Which of the following are measurements of the anteroposterior diameter?
    A. true conjugate
    B. obstetrical conjugate
    C. diagonal conjugate
    D. all of the above   (8:246–7)

106. Which of the following measurements best describes the length of the anterior and posterior walls of the pelvic cavity?

	anterior	posterior
A.	4.5 cm	4.5 to 5 cm
B.	12 cm	12 cm
C.	4.5 to 5 cm	12 cm
D.	12 cm	12 cm

    (8:247)

107. The plane of least pelvic dimensions is that of the
    A. inlet
    B. midpelvis
    C. outlet
    D. none of the above   (5:29)

108. *Major* differences between the male and the female pelvis are due to
    A. heredity
    B. growth hormones
    C. sex hormones
    D. diet   (4:71)

109. In comparing the male and female pelvis, which of the following are characteristic of the female pelvis?
    1. pubic arch has a narrower angle
    2. symphysis is shorter
    3. more shallow
    4. inlet wedge-shaped
    5. inlet heart-shaped

    A. 1, 4
    B. 1, 2, 3
    C. 2, 3, 5
    D. 1, 2, 3, 4   (4:71; 8:257)

110. In considering the mechanical factors associated with the birth process, the mother's pelvis is the
    A. power
    B. passenger
    C. passage
    D. all of the above   (8:243)

111. In considering the passage, which is the most important part of the passenger?
    A. buttocks
    B. shoulder
    C. feet and hands
    D. head   (8:258)

112. In speaking of the relationship between the passenger and the passage, it can be said that during labor there is
    A. an adaptation of the passage to the passenger
    B. an adaptation of the passenger to the passage
    C. no adaptation of either the passage or the passenger
    D. adaptation of both the passage and the passenger   (8:258)

113. The skull is composed of how many bones?
    A. four

B.   six
C.   eight
D.   none of the above   (4:243)

114.   The anterior fontanel closes

   A.   shortly before birth
   B.   shortly after birth
   C.   at about six months
   D.   none of the above   (4:244)

115.   Molding is primarily the process by which

   A.   there is a slight degree of bending of the bones
   B.   there is an overriding of the skull bones at the sutures
   C.   there is a permanent change in the fetal skull
   D.   all of the above   (8:261)

116.   The smallest circumference of the fetal head that passes through the birth canal is at the plane of the

   A.   occipitofrontal diameter
   B.   suboccipitobregmatic diameter
   C.   occipitomental diameter
   D.   biparietal diameter   (8:260)

117.   The largest circumference of the fetal head is at the plane of the

   A.   occipitofrontal diameter
   B.   biparietal diameter
   C.   bitemporal diameter
   D.   occipitomental diameter   (8:260)

118.   When the fetal head enters the pelvis, which of the following diameters (of the fetal head) is usually in the transverse position?

   A.   occipitomental diameter
   B.   biparietal diameter
   C.   suboccipitobregmatic diamter
   D.   none of the above   (8:247)

119.   What percentage of all deliveries are breech presentations?

   A.   3%
   B.   5%
   C.   8%
   D.   10%   (4:244)

120.   The lie of the fetus at term is longitudinal in what percentage of all labors?

   A.   90%
   B.   95%
   C.   99%
   D.   none of the above   (6:235−6)

121.   Sexual maturity in women is evidenced by

   A.   emotional changes
   B.   growth of axillary and pubic hair
   C.   increase in size of external genitalia
   D.   all of the above   (4:85)

122.   Menarche is defined as

   A.   an abnormal flow of menstrual blood
   B.   the cessation of menstrual flow
   C.   the beginning of menstrual flow
   D.   the regular monthly cycle of menstrual flow   (4:685)

123.   Menarche is influenced by

   A.   age
   B.   state of nutrition
   C.   climate
   D.   all of the above   (4:86)

124.   The average age for a girl to have menarche is

   A.   9.5
   B.   11.5
   C.   13.5
   D.   16.5   (2:61)

125.   The irregular menstrual periods that occur following the onset of menses are usually due to

   A.   emotional immaturity of the girl
   B.   physical immaturity of the reproductive system
   C.   failure of ovulation in the girl
   D.   lack of sufficient estrogen in the body   (2:61−2)

126.   Ovulation can best be defined as

   A.   the formation of the corpus luteum
   B.   the growth and discharge of an unimpregnated ovum, usually consistent with the menstrual period
   C.   the rupture of the graafian follicle
   D.   the union of the sperm and ova   (4:686)

127.   Ovulation usually occurs on which of the following days of the usual menstrual cycle?

   A.   first to fourth
   B.   twelfth to sixteenth
   C.   sixteenth to twentieth
   D.   twenty-sixth to twenty-eighth   (8:32)

128.   Menarche is caused by a gradual increase in the production of

   A.   estrogen by the ovary
   B.   gonadotropic hormones by the anterior pituitary gland

C. gonadotropic hormones by the posterior pituitary gland
D. androgen secretions by the adrenal glands (2:61)

129. The usual range of the menstrual cycle, once it is established, is

A. 24 days
B. 28 days
C. 30 days
D. 32 days (2:62)

130. Puberty in the girl best refers to the time at which

A. reproduction becomes possible
B. menstruation begins to take place
C. emotional maturity is complete
D. physical and emotional maturity begin (8:28)

131. Puberty in the boy refers to the time at which

A. spermatozoa make their appearance
B. emotional maturity begins
C. physical maturity is complete
D. emotional and physical maturity begin (8:28)

132. The average age for menarche has decreased by six months in the past decade. This decrease has been attributed to

A. better sex education in the homes, churches, and schools, resulting in less tension regarding menstruation
B. better provisions for physical activities, resulting in better physical conditions in adolescent girls
C. better nutritional standards, resulting in earlier maturation
D. more openness in the younger girl, resulting in more prompt reporting of menarche (2:61)

133. The average amount of blood lost during each menstrual period is

A. 15 mL
B. 25 mL
C. 35 mL
D. 45 mL (2:63)

134. The name given to the phase of the menstrual cycle in which there is a shredding of the endometrial lining of the uterus is

A. progestational phase
B. ovulatory phase
C. menstrual phase
D. secretory phase (8:40)

135. Which phase of the ovulatory cycle corresponds with the proliferative phase of the endometrial cycle?

A. follicular phase
B. ovulatory phase
C. corpus luteum phase
D. none of the above (6:16)

136. Another name for the proliferative phase of the normal menstrual cycle is

A. follicular phase
B. luteal phase
C. premenstrual phase
D. progestational phase (4:89)

137. The shedding of the endometrial lining is due to the regression and the withdrawal of

A. corpus luteum
B. estrogen
C. progesterone
D. all of the above (8:40)

138. Which of the menstrual phases prepares the endometrial lining for pregnancy?

A. luteal phase
B. follicular phase
C. menstrual phase
D. ovulatory phase (8:40)

139. It has been estimated that there are how many immature follicles at birth in every ovary?

A. 100,000
B. 200,000
C. 300,000
D. 400,000 (8:29)

140. The name given to the large number of ova present at birth in the ovary is

A. primary follicle
B. corona radiata
C. primary oocyte
D. zona pellucida (8:29)

141. The female germ cells are found

A. in the medulla portion of the ovary
B. within small follicles in the connective tissue of the cortex
C. between the Sertoli cells
D. none of the above (8:15)

142. The oocytes are produced during the first

A. 12 weeks of fetal life
B. 20 to 24 weeks of fetal life
C. 30 to 32 weeks of fetal life
D. 4 weeks of extrauterine life (8:15)

143. At puberty there are approximately how many ova in each ovary?
    A. 400,000
    B. 200,000
    C. 50,000
    D. 30,000 (8:29)

144. The term "primary follicle" is used to describe
    A. the immature ova or oocyte
    B. the oocyte and the single layer of epithelial cells that surround it
    C. the oocyte and the several layers of epithelial cells that surround it
    D. none of the above (8:29)

145. The hormone estrogen is found in which of the following structures?
    A. theca externa
    B. theca interna
    C. follicular fluid
    D. oocyte (8:30)

146. Who was the first man to see the human ovum through a microscope?
    A. Leeuwenhoek
    B. Ham
    C. de Graaf
    D. von Baer (3:161)

147. Which one of the following is not a gonadotropin produced by the pituitary gland in the female?
    A. follicle-stimulating hormone (FHS)
    B. luteinizing hormone (LH)
    C. interstitial cell-stimulating hormone (ICSH)
    D. lactogenic hormone (LTH) (8:31)

148. Which of the following is an androgen?
    A. progesterone
    B. estrogen
    C. testosterone
    D. luteotropic hormone (8:18)

149. Which of the following is *not* due to the action of estrogen?
    A. breast growth
    B. growth of mild-producing glands and ducts
    C. a feeling of fullness and heaviness in the breasts
    D. none of the above (2:64–5)

150. The luteinizing hormones are responsible for
    A. secretion of breast milk
    B. growth of sex organs
    C. development of vesicular follicles and ovulation
    D. follicular growth (2:63)

151. The term "graafian follicle" is used to describe
    A. the single immature cells scattered throughout the connective tissue of the ovarian cortex
    B. small, spherical bodies in the ovaries, each containing an ovum
    C. the dark-staining, rod-shaped bodies found in the nucleus of cells
    D. none of these (4:684)

152. Who first described the graafian follicle?
    A. van Deventer
    B. de Graaf
    C. Pelty
    D. Mauriceau (4:87)

153. What is the name given to the young male germ cells?
    A. primary spermatocytes
    B. spermatogonia
    C. secondary spermatocytes
    D. spermatids (6:13)

154. Which male germ cells become attached to the Sertoli cells during the developmental stage?
    A. primary spermatocytes
    B. secondary spermatocytes
    C. spermatids
    D. spermatozoa (8:63–4)

155. Which cells are presumed to be responsible for the production of the male sex hormone?
    A. spermatogenic cells
    B. Sertoli's cells
    C. Leydig cells
    D. none of the above (8:20)

156. Where are the spermatozoa stored until they are mature and capable of motility?
    A. seminal vesicle
    B. rete testis
    C. epididymis
    D. seminal duct (8:22)

157. Which of the following produces a secretion that is believed to aid in the neutralization of the acidic vaginal secretions?
    A. prostate gland
    B. bulbourethral glands

C. seminal glands
D. ejaculatory duct (8:23)

158. The testes produce what hormone?

    A. interstitial cell-stimulating hormone
    B. testosterone
    C. diethylstilbestrol
    D. follicle-stimulating hormone (8:24)

159. When conducting fertility tests on men, which one of the following would indicate an unfavorable sperm count?

    A. 100 million/mL
    B. 75 million/mL
    C. 50 million/mL
    D. 20 million/mL (8:24)

160. What percentage of couples in the United States experience difficulty in producing a child?

    A. 5%
    B. 10%
    C. 15%
    D. 20% (3:160)

161. Which of the following factors contribute to a normal couple's ability to conceive?

    1. age of the woman
    2. age of the man
    3. frequency of intercourse
    4. length of exposure

    A. 1, 2, 4
    B. 1, 3, 4
    C. 2, 3, 4
    D. 1, 2, 3, 4 (3:160−1)

162. Menopause usually begins between the ages of

    A. 35 and 40
    B. 40 and 45
    C. 45 and 50
    D. 50 and 55 (2:65)

163. Climacteric means the same as

    A. menopause
    B. ammen
    C. menarche
    D. none of the above (4:93)

164. When menopause approaches there is usually

    A. abrupt amenorrhea
    B. temporary menorrhagia
    C. regularly occurring menses alternating with amenorrhea
    D. none of the above (8:44)

165. "Hot flashes" are believed to be caused by

    1. emotional factors
    2. excessive amounts of follicle-stimulating hormone
    3. decreased amounts of estrogenic hormone
    4. decreased amounts of progesterone
    5. increased amounts of luteinizing hormone

    A. 1, 3
    B. 2, 3
    C. 3, 5
    D. all of the above (8:44)

166. Which of the following alterations in the menstrual cycle pattern is *not* considered as normal?

    A. increased bleeding prior to menopause
    B. prolonged bleeding prior to menopause
    C. bleeding which occurs after menopause
    D. none of the above are considered to be normal (8:44)

167. Which of the following symptoms can be observed in response to the withdrawal of estrogen?

    1. joint pains
    2. headaches
    3. dryness of hair
    4. vasomotor changes
    5. emotional instability

    A. 1, 2, 4
    B. 4, 5
    C. 2, 4, 5
    D. all of the above (4:93−4)

168. Which of the following statements regarding menopause generally seems to hold true?

    A. the earlier the menarche the later the menopause
    B. the earlier the menarche the earlier the menopause
    C. the later the menarche the later the menopause
    D. there appears to be no relationship between menarche and menopause (2:65)

169. What percentage of women experience ill effects as a result of menopause?

    A. 5%
    B. 10%
    C. 15%
    D. none of the above (5:418)

170. Puberty in boys
    A. begins at about the same time as it does in girls
    B. begins about two years later than it does in girls
    C. begins about one year later than it does in girls
    D. none of the above (5:35)

171. A hymenotomy is done to correct
    A. an imperforate anus
    B. an imperforate hymen
    C. lax muscular structure of the vagina
    D. none of these (2:54)

172. Which of the following are *not* due to the action of progesterone?
    1. causes a rise in basal temperature
    2. inhibits contractions of the uterus
    3. causes an increase in the size of the uterus
    4. promotes secretory changes in the endometrium
    5. produces enlargement of the labia minora

    A. 1, 2
    B. 2, 4
    C. 3, 5
    D. none of the above (2:64)

173. In what percentage of couples is it impossible to find a medical reason for infertility?
    A. 3 to 5%
    B. 5 to 10%
    C. 10 to 15%
    D. 15 to 18% (3:161)

174. Approximately how long should a couple attempt to conceive a child before seeking medical advice?
    A. 6 months
    B. 1 year
    C. 18 months
    D. 2 years (4:131)

175. Which of the following signs are present at the time of ovulation?
    1. pH of cervical mucus 7.0
    2. cervical mucus forms threads 1 to 2 in. long
    3. cervical mucus forms cellular pattern
    4. luteal phase of menstrual cycle
    5. body temperature remains stable

    A. 1, 3, 4
    B. 2, 3, 5
    C. all of the above
    D. none of the above (8:33,38,40)

176. Dysmenorrhea is caused by
    A. tension
    B. anxiety
    C. emotional states
    D. none of these (2:654)

177. Which of the following measures will probably *not* provide relief from dysmenorrhea?
    A. good posture
    B. cold baths
    C. rest and quiet
    D. heat to lumbar region (8:42)

178. Menorrhagia in adolescents is usually due to
    A. genetic abnormalities
    B. pelvic abnormality
    C. hormonal imbalance
    D. nutritional deficiency (2:654)

179. The pubic hair is called
    A. espalier
    B. escutcheon
    C. erose
    D. none of the above (6:3)

180. Which of the following is considered to be a function of the vagina?
    A. the canal through which the menstrual flow escapes
    B. the female organ of sexual union
    C. the birth canal during delivery
    D. all of the above (5:18)

181. Testicular functioning in men
    A. stops between the ages of 35 and 45
    B. continues until the age of 50
    C. is active until the age of 60
    D. does not stop at a definite age (8:22)

182. At the time of ovulation, the cervical mucus forms a fern-like pattern called
    A. spinnbarkheit
    B. arborization
    C. mittelschmerz
    D. none of the above (8:39)

Directions: Each group of numbered words or phrases is followed by a list of lettered statements. MATCH the lettered statement with the numbered word or phrase most closely associated with it.

Questions 183 through 186

183. painful menstruation
184. excessive amount of menstrual flow
185. bleeding between periods
186. absence of menstruation

A. menorrhagia
B. dysmenorrhea
C. amenorrhea
D. metorrhagia   (8:42)

Questions 187 through 190
187. oocyte grows in size; follicular fluid develops and forms vesicle; occurs from puberty until menopause
188. oocyte undergoes cytolysis; follicular fluid absorbs; occurs from fetal life until after menopause
189. oocyte and follicular fluid extruded; occurs for about 8 days each month
190. oocyte and follicular fluid extruded; occurs for about 12 weeks

A. corpus luteum of menstruation
B. corpus luteum of pregnancy
C. follicular atresia
D. graafian follicle   (8:30−5)

Questions 191 through 194
191. female germ cell during period of immaturity
192. female germ cell surrounded by primordial follicle
193. female germ cell before meiosis
194. female germ cell after meiosis and before development of the ovum

A. ootid
B. oocyte
C. primary oocyte
D. oogonium   (6:15)

Questions 195 through 198
195. hormone responsible for beginning of formation of corpus luteum
196. hormone responsible for maintaining corpus luteum
197. hormone responsible for proliferative phase in the endometrium
198. hormone responsible for the stimulation of the glands that secrete mucin and glycogen

A. progesterone
B. estrogen

C. luteinizing homrone
D. luteotropic hormone   (6:15−6)

Questions 199 through 202
199. substance produced by seminal vesicle
200. substance produced by Leydig cells
201. substance produced by pituitary gland
202. substance produced by spermatogenic cells

A. testosterone
B. prostaglandin
C. ICSH
D. spermatozoa   (6:61;8:21)

Questions 203 through 206
203. diagonal conjugate
204. interspinous
205. intertuberous
206. posterior sagittal

A. 12.5
B. 11
C. 7.5
D. 10.5   (8:252−3)

Questions 207 through 210
207. junction between last lumbar vertebra and sacrum
208. junction between sacrum and coccyx
209. junction between two pubic bones
210. junction between sacrum and ilium

A. sacrococcygeal articulation
B. sacral promontory
C. sacroiliac articulation
D. symphysis pubis   (4:66−7)

Questions 211 through 214
211. suture that runs between two frontal bones
212. suture that extends anteroposteriorly between the parietal bones
213. suture that lies between frontal bones and anterior margin of the parietals
214. suture that separates posterior margins of parietals from upper margin of the occipital bone

A. coronal
B. frontal
C. sagittal
D. lambdoidal   (8:259)

Answers and Explanations:
Anatomy and Physiology of the Female and Male Reproductive Systems

1. **C.** Occasionally the term "pudendum" is used to describe this group of organs.

2. **C.** These organs are: the mons veneris, labia majora, labia minora, clitoris, hymen, vestibule, and various glands.

3. **A.** After puberty this organ is covered with hair.

4. **A.** The vestibule becomes visible when the labia minora are spread apart.

5. **C.** The urinary meatus is not part of the external genitalia but is included because of its anatomic location.

6. **C.** The vaginal orifice is partly covered by the hymen.

7. **B.** The labia minora are situated between the labia majora with their outer surfaces in contact with the labia majora.

8. **B.** Although the labia majora usually lie in close opposition to each other, they may gape in the multigravidae.

9. **C.** Anteriorly, the labia minora join together to form a double ridge of tissue. The ridge above the clitoris is termed the prepuce.

10. **D.** There are no glands in the vagina.

11. **B.** The Bartholin's glands are found at the base of the labia majora.

12. **B.** The Skene's glands in women are located on either side of the urethra.

13. **B.** If these veins are not properly repaired during delivery they can hemorrhage.

14. **B.** The fornix is the upper end of the vagina; it forms a circular cuff around the cervix.

15. **C.** When stimulated in sex play, the clitoris becomes engorged with blood and thus becomes more erect. The tiny nerve endings become increasingly sensitive to erotic stimulation and may produce an orgasm.

16. **C.** The perineal body fills the wedge-shaped area between the lower ends of the rectum and vagina and forms a central attachment for the muscle and fascia of the pelvic floor.

17. **C.** The pelvic diaphragm stretches across the lowermost part of the pelvic cavity.

18. **D.** All of the statements represent functions of the pelvic diaphragm.

19. **B.** Both of these muscles are actually paired muscles. The levator ani stretches from the pubic bones to the spine of the ischial bones, and the coccygeus muscles arise at the ischial spines and insert into the coccyx and lower part of the sacrum.

20. **A.** In obstetrical practice, the term "perineum" is used to refer to the area between the fourchette and the anus.

21. **B.** The perineum is made of the bulbocavernosus, the transverse perineal muscles, and also those muscles forming the anal sphincters.

22. **B.** Before the birth of a child, the external os is a small round opening. Following the birth of a child, it is converted into a small transverse opening. Carunculae myrtiforms are the remnants of the hymen present after childbirth. Lacerations of the perineal tissue are most often the result of childbirth.

23. **C.** The pH of the cervical mucus is about 7.5 at the time of ovulation.

24. **D.** The diameter of the cervix is approximately 1 in.

25. **D.** The cervix is about one third the length of the corpus.

26. **B.** The fossa navicularis is the shallow depression located between the fourchette and the vaginal orifice.

27. **C.** The cul-de-sac of Douglas separates the lower part of the uterus from the rectum.

28. **B.** The perineum is made up of muscles and fascia and supports the pelvic structures.

29. **B.** The vaginal secretions during the childbearing years are normally acid, with a pH from 4.0 to 5.0.

30. **B.** Colporrhaphy is any operation during which the vagina is sutured.

31. **C.** The breasts are considered to be accessory organs of reproduction because they undergo many physiologic changes during pregnancy.

32. **C.** There are about 15 to 20 lobes in each breast. These lobes are arranged radially around the nipple.

33. **B.** There are about 15 to 20 small openings of the lactiferous ducts at the nipple tip.

34. **B.** The pudendal artery is one of the chief suppliers of blood to the perineum.

35. **C.** The chief source of the blood supply to the perineum is the inferior hemorrhoidal and pudendal arteries.

36. **C.** Nerve innervation to the breast comes from the fourth, fifth, and sixth thoracic nerves and also from the supraclavicular nerves.

37. **B.** In the adult woman, the breasts weigh between 100 and 200 g.

38. **B.** The circular area in the center of the breast is called the areola. The pigmentation varies with functional changes from pink to brownish-red.

39. **B.** The nipple is also called the mammary papilla.

40. **C.** The nipple contains fibromuscular tissue that becomes erectile on stimulation from the child's sucking during lactation.

41. **C.** These sacs or alveoli are lined with a single layer of cells that secrete milk.

42. **D.** The clitoris is an external organ and thus part of the vulva.

43. **C.** The uterus is also the organ from which menstruation occurs.

44. **B.** The endometrium, or innermost layer, is shed during the menstrual flow. The middle layer is the muscular layer, and the outer layer is known as the perimetrium.

45. **C.** The largest amount of blood goes to the uterus through the uterine arteries, which are branches of the hypogastric arteries. A smaller amount of blood reaches the uterus from the ovarian arteries, which are branches of the aorta.

46. **C.** The muscle fibers in the fundus have the power of great retractability and contractability.

47. **C.** The softening of the isthmus of the uterus is a probable sign of pregnancy and called Hegar's sign.

48. **D.** The muscle tissue of the uterus is nonstriated, or smooth.

49. **B.** The nerve supply to the uterus is derived primarily from the sympathetic nervous system. However, the cerebrospinal and parasympathetic systems also play a part.

50. **B.** The cardinal or Mackenrodt's ligaments provide the chief support for the uterus.

51. **B.** The uterosacral ligaments aid in keeping the uterus in its normal position by exerting traction on the cervix.

52. **D.** These are all functions of the ovary.

53. **D.** All of the factors mentioned can be attributed to the functions of the ovary.

54. **B.** The inner layer of the ovary is called the medulla.

55. **B.** The ovaries are suspended by folds of peritoneum called mesovarium.

56. **B.** The fimbria ovarica, one of the fimbria, has the form of a shallow goiter and extends close to the ovary and picks up the ova that is expelled from the ovary.

57. **D.** It is also called the fimbriated end because of the large number of fine fringes that cover this portion of the fallopian tube.

58. **B.** The length of the fallopian tube varies from 7 to 14 in. each.

59. **C.** The fallopian tubes are lined with mucous membrane, which lies in longitudinal folds. This membrane contains ciliated epithelium.

60. **D.** All of the nerves mentioned supply both the uterus and the fallopian tubes.

61. **D.** All three occurrences aid the fallopian tube in its primary function—that of transporting the ovum to the uterus.

62. **B.** The testes produce germ cells (spermatozoa and testosterone, a male hormone).

63. **A.** The testes are the sex organs of the male.

64. **B.** In addition to functioning as a part of the long excretory duct from the testes, the vas deferens serves as a storage site for sperm.

65. **C.** The internal organs of the male reproductive system are the testes and a canal system with accessory glands.

66. **B.** The vas deferens is part of the canal system.

67. **B.** The narrow, coiled tubules within each testis are called seminiferous tubules.

68. **B.** The testes usually descend through the inguinal canal and into the scrotum during the seventh or eighth month of fetal life.

69. **C.** The combined length of the many seminiferous tubules in one testis equals almost a mile.

70. **B.** In men, the germinal epithelium or spermatogenic cells continue to produce immature germ cells during sexual maturity.

71. **B.** Sperm remain in the epididymis for approximately 18 hours, during which time they become motile and capable of fertilizing an ovum.

72. **A.** The arteries and veins form a part of the spermatic cords.

73. **C.** The vas deferentia are bilateral ducts approximately 18 in. long.

74. **B.** The pH of semen varies from 7.35 to 7.50.

75. **C.** The glans penis contains the urethral opening and many very sensitive nerve endings.

76. **D.** The fetus begins its entrance into the world through the bony pelvis, and the normal female pelvis is constructed to facilitate its passage.

77. **D.** The coccyx forms the terminal end of the vertebral column.

78. **A.** The articulation that joins the two hip bones in the front of the pelvis is called the symphysis pubis.

79. **B.** During delivery, the coccyx is forced backward 1 in. or more through the action of the sacrococcygeal joint.

80. **C.** The sacrum is a wedge-shaped bone formed by the fusion of five vertebrae. The sacral promontory is the upper anterior portion, which is formed by the junction of the last vertebra with the sacrum.

81. **D.** This increased mobility is due to the action of relaxin, an ovarian hormone.

82. **D.** The false pelvis also offers some landmarks that are important for the practice of pelvimetry.

83. **C.** The ilium is part of the false pelvis and thus not part of the true pelvis.

84. **B.** During labor, the baby's head enters the pelvic inlet with its longest diameter in the transverse (side-to-side) diameter of the pelvis.

85. **B.** The baby's head, during labor, thus descends in a straight line until it reaches the ischial spines and then curves forward toward the pelvic outlet.

86. **A.** The baby's head exits from the outlet with its largest diameter in the anterior-posterior position (front to back).

87. **B.** The linea terminalis bounds the area called the inlet (or pelvic brim).

88. **D.** Complete ossification takes place at this time.

89. **C.** The gynecoid pelvis is the best one for childbearing.

90. **D.** The safe passage of the full-term baby through the pelvis is the primary goal of obstetrics.

91. **C.** X-ray pelvimetry can measure the diameters of the pelvis and also the relationship of the term baby to the pelvis.

92. **D.** Ischial diameter is the distance between the ischial tuberosities, thus the transverse diameter of the outlet.

93. **A.** The diagonal conjugate is the distance between the sacral promontory and the undersurface of the symphysis pubis.

94. **B.** In order to obtain the distance between the sacral promontory and the posterior aspect of the symphysis pubis (the conjugate vera), 1.5 cm is deducted from the measurement of the diameter of the diagonal conjugate.

95. **A.** The true conjugate should be about 11 cm.

96. **D.** The intertuberous diameter is the shortest diameter of the pelvic outlet. A diameter of 8 cm or more is considered normal.

97. **A.** The anteroposterior diameter of the outlet extends from the middle of the lower margin of the symphysis pubis to the tip of the sacrum.

98. **B.** The posterior sagittal diameter is the distance from the midpoint of an imaginary line between the ischial tuberosities to the sacrum.

99. **B.** The lower end of the ischium is known as the ischial tuberosities. The body rests upon these two projections when in a sitting position.

100. **C.** The ischial spines are located in the posterior borders of the ischium.

101. **B.** The inlet of the pelvis is at a 50- to 60-degree angle with the horizontal.

102. **B.** The pubic arch is the portion of the true pelvis extending from one ischial tuberosity to the other.

103. **B.** These areas of articulation are called the sacroiliac joints.

104. **B.** Transverse diameter is the greatest diameter between the linea terminalis on each side of the inlet and measures 13 cm or slightly less.

105. **D.** The true conjugate is the distance between the top of the symphysis pubis and the middle of the sacral promontory and usually measures 11 cm or slightly more. The obstetrical conjugate is the distance between the inner surface of the symphysis pubis and the sacral promontory and usually measures several millimeters less than the true conjugate. The diagonal conjugate is the distance between the lower margin of the symphysis pubis and the sacral promontory and is from 1.5 to 2 cm larger than the true conjugate.

106. **C.** The posterior wall of the pelvic cavity is formed by the sacrum, and the anterior wall is formed by the symphysis pubis.

107. **B.** Here, the anteroposterior diameter, which extends from the lower margin of the symphysis pubis to the sacrum, measures 11.5 cm, and the transverse diameter, which extends between the ischial spines, measures 10.5 cm.

108. **C.** The major differences between the male and female pelvis appear at puberty and are therefore due to the influence of the sex hormones.

109. **C.** In addition to those characteristics listed, the most conspicuous difference is that in women the pubic arch is much wider.

110. **C.** The mother's pelvis is referred to as the passage.

111. **D.** The fetal head is usually the part of the body that passes through the birth canal first and is the largest and most malleable part.

112. **B.** During labor there is a series of changes in the size, shape, and position of the fetal head in relation to the size and shape of the maternal pelvis.

113. **C.** The skull is made up of eight bones. Four of these bones—sphenoid, ethmoid, and two temporal bones—lie at the base of the cranium. The four bones that form the upper portion of the cranium are the frontal, occipital, and two parietal bones.

114. **D.** The anterior fontanel closes when the child is slightly over a year old.

115. **B.** The fetal skull is made up of individual bones separated by soft membranous spaces. Compression against the head results in the overriding of the skull bones.

116. **B.** The suboccipitobregmatic circumference is measured around from below the occipital protuberance to the center of the anterior fontanelle or bregma and is 32 cm.

117. **A.** The occipitofrontal circumference is measured around from the occipital protuberance to a point above the birdge of the nose and is about 34.5 cm.

118. **C.** The suboccipitobregmatic diameter is measured from the undersurface of the occiput where it joins the neck to the center of the anterior fontanel and is 9.5 cm.

119. **A.** The breech presentation occurs in about 3% of all cases.

120. **C.** The lie (relation of the long axis of the fetus to the long axis of the mother) is longitudinal in 99% of all labors.

121. **D.** At the time of puberty, evidence of sexual maturity in the young woman is evidenced by both bodily and emotional changes.

122. **C.** There are usually dramatic bodily changes prior to the onset of menarche.

123. **D.** Heredity and environment may also influence the early or late appearance of menarche.

124. **B.** Menarche usually begins between the ages of 9 and 13. The average age is 11.5 years.

125. **C.** If ovulation is not occurring, there is no progesterone secretion, and thus the rhythm of the cycle is often disturbed.

126. **B.** Ovulation is referred to as the growth and discharge of an unimpregnated ovum, usually consistent with the menstrual period.

127. **B.** The time of ovulation is approximately 14 days before the end of the cycle, which means

about 14 days before the first day of the next menstrual period.

128. **B.** At adolescence, the anterior pituitary gland begins to secrete gonadotropic hormones, which in turn gradually stimulate the gonads to produce hormones and to mature germ cells.

129. **B.** The range of the menstrual cycle in normal women may be as short as 20 days or as long as 45 days.

130. **B.** In girls, the appearance of the first menstrual period is commonly accepted as evidence of puberty.

131. **A.** In boys, puberty is defined as the time when spermatozoa make their appearance.

132. **C.** Experts attribute the decreased age for menarche to better nutrition and thus an earlier maturation.

133. **C.** During the menstrual flow approximately 35 mL of blood and 35 mL of serous fluid and desquamated tissue are lost per month.

134. **C.** The menstrual phase is a period of regression during which the well-developed endometrium becomes ischemic, degenerates, and desquamates with moderate bleeding.

135. **A.** The follicular phase of the ovulatory cycle (day 1 to 12) corresponds with the proliferative phase of the endometrial cycle.

136. **A.** Each month estrogen stimulates the endometrium to be built up. This phase is called both the proliferative and follicular phase.

137. **D.** The menstrual phase coincides with regression of the corpus luteum and withdrawal of its hormones, progesterone and estrogen.

138. **A.** By the end of the luteal phase, the endometrium is soft, velvety, and edematous and measures 4 to 6 cm in thickness. It is ready for implantation and nourishment of a fertilized ovum.

139. **B.** It has been estimated that at birth each ovary contains 200,000 (or even more) immature follicles.

140. **C.** The primary oocytes are present in the ovary at birth and probably provide the woman with ova for life.

141. **B.** The female germ cells are found within small follicles in the connective tissue of the cortex.

142. **B.** The germ cells in women are produced during the first 20 to 24 weeks of fetal life. After this time there is no further development of the female germ cell.

143. **C.** By puberty there are about 50,000 ova remaining in each ovary.

144. **B.** At birth each oocyte (or ovum) is surrounded by a single layer of flattened cells.

145. **C.** The follicular fluid is found in the center of the graafian follicle and contains the hormone estrogen.

146. **D.** Karl Ernst von Baer saw the first ovum in 1827.

147. **B.** This hormone may be called the intersitital cell-stimulating hormone in men because of its stimulating effect on the interstitial cells in the testes to produce testosterone.

148. **C.** An androgen is any substance that possesses masculinizing activities, such as the testes hormone, testosterone.

149. **C.** Progesterone causes the breasts to feel full and heavy (during the nonpregnant state).

150. **C.** The developing vesicular follicles that do not ovulate atrophy either before or immediately after ovulation occurs.

151. **B.** The bodies or vesicles contain the follicular fluid and the ovum.

152. **B.** Reijnier de Graaf, the Dutch physician, first described the graafian follicle in 1672.

153. **B.** The young male germ cells are called spermatogonia.

154. **C.** The spermatids become attached to the Sertoli cells that are present in the lining of the seminiferous tubules. Here they gradually develop into spermatozoa.

155. **C.** The Leydig or interstitial cells are located in the framework of connective tissue between the seminiferous tubules.

156. **C.** The spermatozoa are retained in the epididymides for about three weeks.

157. **B.** Bulbourethral glands, or Cowper's glands, are two small pea-sized bodies located below the prostate glands, within the pelvic floor.

158. **B.** The testes serve as an endocrine gland producing a typically male hormone called testosterone.

159. **D.** A count of 20 million or less sperm per milliliter is considered to be unfavorable for fertilization. The normal count is 50 to 150 million spermatozoa per milliliter of semen.

160. **C.** These couples are either infertile or sterile.

161. **D.** All of the factors mentioned contribute generally to a normal couple's ability to conceive.

162. **C.** The usual age among American women is 47 years.

163. **D.** The terms "menopause" and "climacteric" are often used synonymously. However, "menopause" refers to the cessation of menstruation, whereas "climacteric" is defined as the syndrome of endocrine, somatic, and psychic changes occurring at the termination of the reproductive period in women.

164. **C.** Menstruation gradually ceases as menopause approaches.

165. **B.** A decrease in ovarian functioning disturbs the relationship between pituitary gonadotropic and ovarian hormone production. Vasomotor changes may be the result of either statement 2 or 3.

166. **D.** Any of the menstrual cycle patterns mentioned may be indicative of a problem and should be called to the attention of the physician.

167. **D.** All of the symptoms mentioned can be observed in a woman during menopause.

168. **A.** In general, menopause tends to occur earlier among women who had a late menarche, and later among women who had an early menarche.

169. **D.** Approximately 25% of all women have severe enough ill effects to warrant medical attention.

170. **C.** Puberty in boys begins about one year later than in girls. Any age between 10 and 16 is within normal range.

171. **B.** In an imperforate hymen, the hymen covers the vaginal opening with a thick, tough membrane. Surgical opening through the hymen is termed "hymenotomy".

172. **C.** Enlargement of the labia minora and increase in the size of the uterus are caused by the action of estrogen.

173. **B.** In 5 to 10% of all cases of infertility it is impossible to find any medical reason for the problem.

174. **B.** If a couple have tried for a year to conceive a child without results, then medical help should be sought.

175. **D.** At ovulation, the cervical mucus has a pH of near 7.5, can be drawn from the vagina in threads of 15 to 20 cm in length, and forms complete fern-like patterns. Ovulation occurs between the follicular and luteal phase of the menstrual cycle, and there is a rise in temperature at the time of ovulation.

176. **D.** The specific cause of dysmenorrhea is unknown.

177. **B.** Cold baths during periods of dysmenorrhea will probably increase discomfort rather than decrease it.

178. **C.** Menorrhagia in the adolescent girl is usually caused by hormonal imbalance. This problem should correct itself in several years.

179. **B.** The pubic hair is called escutcheon.

180. **D.** All of the points listed are considered to be functions of the vagina.

181. **D.** Testicular functioning in men does not show a sharp decline or stoppage at any particular age.

182. **B.** Arborization, or the fern pattern, is dependent upon estrogen stimulation; thus the presence of arborization indicates that ovulation has taken place.

183. **B.** Dysmenorrhea is painful menstruation.

184. **A.** Menorrhagia is excessive menstrual flow.

185. **D.** Metorrhagia is bleeding between menstrual periods.

186. **C.** Amenorrhea is absence of menstruation.

187. **D.** A graafian follicle is a vesicle whose activity extends from puberty until menopause.

188. **C.** Follicular atresia is a process by which the primary oocytes degenerate without rupture and thus disappear from within the uterus.

189. **A.** The corpus luteum of menstruation persists for about eight days, after which secretory activity decreases, menstruation begins in about eight days, and regression of the corpus luteum is soon complete.

190. **B.** The corpus luteum of pregnancy persists for about 12 weeks. The placenta begins production of the corpus luteum hormones at a very early stage of development and by the end of three months takes over this role from the corpus luteum.

191. **D.** Oogonium is the name given to the female germ cell prior to its process of maturation.

192. **B.** Oocytes (primitive ova) is the name given to the female germ cells during the early time they are surrounded by the primordial follicle.

193. **C.** Primary oocyte is the name given to the female germ cells immediately prior to meiosis.

194. **A.** Ootid is the name given to the female germ cell that becomes the ovum following meiosis.

195. **C.** The luteinizing hormone stimulates ovulation and thus the beginning of corpus luteum formation.

196. **D.** The luteotropic hormone stimulates luteal cells to produce progesterone, and thus it maintains the corpus luteum.

197. **B.** Estrogen is responsible for the marked growth of the glands and stroma of the endometrium.

198. **A.** Progesterone stimulates the glands of the endometrium to secrete mucin and glycogen.

199. **B.** The seminal vesicle secretes prostaglandin.

200. **A.** The Leydig cells produce testosterone.

201. **C.** The pituitary gland secretes interstitial cell-stimulating hormone.

202. **D.** The spermatogenic cells produce spermatozoa.

203. **A.** The average length of the diagonal conjugage is about 12.5 cm.

204. **D.** The average length of the interspinous diameter is 10.5 cm.

205. **B.** The average length of the intertuberous diameter is 11 cm.

206. **C.** The average length of the posterior sagittal is 7.5 cm.

207. **B.** The projection formed by the junction of the last lumbar vertebra with the sacrum is known as the sacral promontory.

208. **A.** The junction between the sacrum and the coccyx is called the sacrococcygeal articulation.

209. **D.** The junction between the two pubic bones is called the symphysis pubis.

210. **C.** The junction between the sacrum and the ilium on either side of the pelvis is called the sacroiliac articulation.

211. **B.** The frontal suture lies between the two frontal bones.

212. **C.** The sagittal suture extends anteroposteriorly between the parietal bones.

213. **A.** The coronal suture lies between the frontal bones and the anterior margin of the parietals.

214. **D.** The lambdoidal suture separates the posterior margins of the parietals from the upper margin of the occipital bone.

CHAPTER 3

Physiology and Development of the Fetus

At the time of conception a new life begins. From this point until the occurrence of childbirth, a host of specific factors will affect and determine the course of fetal development.

The material in this chapter covers germ cell development and maturation and the effect of internal forces on the developing child within the uterus.

Directions: Each of the questions or incomplete statements below is followed by four suggested answers or completions. Select the BEST answer in each case.

1. The human cell contains how many chromosomes?
   A. 22
   B. 23
   C. 44
   D. 46   (8:49)

2. The division of chromosomes in the human cell is
   A. 44 autosomes and 2 sex chromosomes
   B. 43 autosomes and 1 sex chromosome
   C. 22 pairs of autosomes and 1 pair of sex chromosomes
   D. 21 pairs of autosomes and 1 pair of sex chromosomes   (4:96)

3. The mature human ovum prior to fertilization contains how many chromosomes?
   A. 22
   B. 23
   C. 44
   D. 46   (4:96)

4. The male cells contain
   A. one X and one Y chromosome
   B. two X chromosomes
   C. two Y chromosomes
   D. no sex chromosomes   (4:96)

5. How many groups of chromosomes are there?
   A. three
   B. five
   C. seven
   D. nine   (8:51)

6. Which of the following chromosome combinations will produce a baby girl?
   A. XX
   B. XY
   C. YY
   D. YX   (5:44)

7. The nucleus of the sperm contains how many chromosomes?
   A. 23
   B. 24
   C. 46
   D. 48   (6:75)

8. Immediately after the union of the male and female pronucleus, the ovum contains how many chromosomes?
   A. 23
   B. 46
   C. 47
   D. 48   (6:75)

9. During meiosis, the number of chromosomes
   A. is doubled
   B. is divided by one half

C. is tripled
D. remains the same (4:96)

10. A chromosome is

A. a germinal factor that carries on a hereditary transmissible character
B. a dark-staining, rod-shaped body
C. a tumor found by malignant proliferation of the epithelium of the chorionic villi
D. none of these (8:49−52)

11. The description of an individual in terms of the kinds of genes he has in respect to a given characteristic is the

A. karyotype
B. genotype
C. phenotype
D. none of the above (8:52)

12. Prior to ovulation, the ovum undergoes a process termed

A. mitosis
B. meiosis
C. cleavage
D. none of the above (4:95)

13. During transport to the uterus, the ovum is suspended in

A. liquor folliculi
B. cytoplasm
C. liquor amni
D. vesicular fluid (6:15)

14. The process by which sperm are ejaculated into the vagina is called

A. fertilization
B. semination
C. fecundation
D. none of the above (6:75)

15. The fusion of the sperm and the ovum is called

A. fecundation
B. conception
C. impregnation
D. all of the above (6:75)

16. Penetration of the sperm into the ovum is aided by the action of

A. proteolytic enzymes
B. hyaluronidase
C. cytolytic enzymes
D. none of the above (8:76)

17. Following ovulation, the ovum remains viable for a period of approximately

A. 1 to 2 hours
B. 3 to 6 hours
C. 12 hours
D. 24 hours (8:76)

18. Sperm may remain viable for

A. 2 to 4 hours
B. 4 to 8 hours
C. 24 to 48 hours
D. 72 hours (8:76)

19. At the time of ejaculation, approximately how many spermatozoa are discharged into the vagina?

A. 100 million
B. 200 million
C. 300 million
D. 400 million (4:102)

20. Fertilization usually occurs in the

A. uterus
B. vagina
C. medial portion of the fallopian tubes
D. distal portion of the fallopian tubes (5:45)

21. Movement of the fertilized ovum through the fallopian tube is accomplished by

A. ciliary current within the tube
B. muscular contractions within the tube
C. both A and B
D. none of the above (5:46)

22. The "zygote" is another term for the

A. ovum
B. developing embryo
C. ovaries
D. spermatozoa (8:77)

23. What percentage of all twins is identical?

A. 11%
B. 33%
C. 67%
D. 80% (6:65)

24. Fertilization of one ovum may result in which of the following types of pregnancies?

1. one male child
2. one female child
3. two male children
4. one male and one female child
5. monozygotic twins

A. 1, 2
B. 1, 2, 3

C.   1, 2, 4
D.   1, 2, 3, 5   (8:92)

25. Triplets may be the result of
     A.   one ovum
     B.   two ova
     C.   three ova
     D.   all of the above   (8:92—3)

26. As the zygote moves through the fallopian tube, it becomes a solid ball of cells called the
     A.   trophoblast
     B.   blastocyst
     C.   morula
     D.   none of the above   (4:104)

27. The process of nidation takes
     A.   3 days
     B.   7 days
     C.   10 days
     D.   14 days   (6:76)

28. At the time of implantation, the embryo is called a
     A.   zygote
     B.   ·morula
     C.   blastocyst
     D.   cytotrophoblast   (8:80)

29. At implantation, the endometrium is in what menstrual phase?
     A.   proliferative
     B.   secretory
     C.   menstrual
     D.   follicular   (4:88—9)

30. What is the name given to the endometrium during pregnancy?
     A.   chorion
     B.   decidua
     C.   peritoneum
     D.   none of the above   (4:107)

31. Implantation of the ovum into the uterine wall is accomplished through the action of
     A.   embryoblasts
     B.   trophoblasts
     C.   blastomeres
     D.   none of the above   (8:79)

32. Implantation of the fertilized ovum in the uterine lining occurs approximately how many days after conception?
     A.   3
     B.   4

C.   7
D.   11   (8:80)

33. The decidua reaches its maximum height at about what period of the pregnancy?
     A.   at time of implantation of the ovum
     B.   at the third or fourth month of pregnancy
     C.   at the eighth month of pregnancy
     D.   at term   (8:82)

34. What is the name of the hormone produced by the placenta which causes lactational changes in mammary tissue and produces growth-like effect?
     A.   chorionic gonadotropin
     B.   chorionic thyrotropin
     C.   chorionic somatomammotropin
     D.   none of the above   (6:83—4)

35. Which of the following cells secrete progesterone?
     A.   cytotrophoblastic cells
     B.   syncytial cells (of the trophoblasts)
     C.   Sertoli cells
     D.   theca interna   (6:83)

36. Which hormone stimulates the corpus luteum to be continued?
     A.   estrogen
     B.   chorionic gonadotropin
     C.   FSH
     D.   posterior pituitary gland   (8:89)

37. Which hormone provides the basis for the pregnancy tests?
     A.   progesterone
     B.   chorionic gonadotropin
     C.   prolactin hormone
     D.   none of the above   (8:89)

38. Which of the following hormones is *not* produced by the placenta?
     A.   estrogen
     B.   chorionic gonadotropin
     C.   progesterone
     D.   interstitial cell-stimulating hormone
                                       (8:89)

39. The amniotic fluid comes in direct contact with
     A.   the chorion
     B.   the amnion
     C.   the decidua capsularis
     D.   none of the above   (8:83)

40. Which of the following are considered to be functions of the amniotic fluid?
    1. fetal metabolism
    2. provision of movement for the fetus
    3. protection from possible injury for the fetus
    4. provision of uniform temperature for the fetus
    5. acts as water wedge during labor
    A. 2, 3, 4
    B. 1, 2, 3, 4
    C. 2, 3, 4, 5
    D. all of the above   (8:83−4)

41. Approximately how much amniotic fluid does the fetus swallow per day by the time it reaches term?
    A. 50 mL
    B. 100 mL
    C. 300 mL
    D. 450 mL   (8:83)

42. The largest amount of amniotic fluid is present in the uterus during which of the following time periods?
    A. end of sixth month
    B. end of eighth month
    C. at term
    D. immediately before rupture of the membranes   (2:100)

43. The pH of the amniotic fluid is about
    A. 6.2
    B. 7.2
    C. 4.6
    D. 4.8   (6:79)

44. What percentage of the amniotic fluid is replaced every hour in the latter part of pregnancy?
    A. 5%
    B. 15%
    C. 35%
    D. 50%   (6:79)

45. Which of the following sets of structures arise from the entoderm germ layer?
    A. nasal passages, nervous system, skin, and appendages
    B. alimentary canal, lungs, liver, and bladder
    C. reproductive organs, circulatory system, and bones
    D. anus, external ear, and muscles (8:81)

46. During the first eight weeks or so, the developing organism is called the
    A. embryo
    B. fetus
    C. zygote
    D. none of the above   (8:82)

47. Which structure is the forerunner of the umbilical cord?
    A. yolk sac
    B. allantois
    C. body stalk
    D. chorionic villi   (8:90)

48. The average length of the umbilical cord is
    A. 30 cm
    B. 55 cm
    C. 75 cm
    D. 100 cm   (8:90)

49. Researchers have indicated that the purpose of Wharton's jelly is
    A. to protect the umbilical cord from the effects of the alkaline amniotic fluid
    B. to inhibit bleeding from the umbilical cord stump following delivery
    C. to protect the cord from injury during intrauterine existence
    D. not clearly known   (6:77)

50. The umbilical cord consists of which of the following?
    A. one artery, two veins, and Wharton's jelly
    B. two arteries, one vein, and Wharton's jelly
    C. two arteries, two veins, and Wharton's jelly
    D. none of the above   (8:92)

51. Blood is carried from the fetus to the placenta through the
    A. umbilical artery
    B. umbilical vein
    C. two umbilical arteries
    D. two umbilical veins   (4:117)

52. Approximately how much blood flows through the cord every minute?
    A. one-quarter pint
    B. one-half pint
    C. one pint
    D. two pints   (6:77)

53. The rule used to determine the week of gestation of a fetus by measurement of its length is
    A. Nagele's rule
    B. Haase's rule
    C. Bartholin's rule
    D. none of these   (5:51)

54. The average length of pregnancy from time of conception is
    A. 300 days
    B. 266 days
    C. 280 days
    D. 320 days   (4:114)

55. Maturity in the fetus can be determined by
    A. ultrasonic estimate, which indicates a biparietal diameter of less than 8.7 cm
    B. concentration of 2 mg/dL creatinine in amniotic fluid sample
    C. fat cells less than 2% of total cells present in amniotic fluid sample
    D. presence of bilirubin in sample of amniotic fluid   (6:95)

56. Growth and development in the embryo
    A. proceeds at an even pace in all parts of the developing organs
    B. occurs first in the upper parts of the organism and then in lower parts
    C. occurs first in the lower parts of the organism and then in the upper parts
    D. none of the above   (5:46−7)

57. The time of fertilization can be fairly reliably calculated to be
    A. first day after the onset of the last menstrual period
    B. seventh day after the onset of last menstrual period
    C. fourteenth day after the onset of last menstrual period
    D. cannot be known   (8:96)

58. The majority of body systems in the embryo have begun to develop by the end of the
    A. second week
    B. third week
    C. fourth week
    D. sixth week   (8:97)

59. The fetal heart is functioning by the end of
    A. third week
    B. fourth week
    C. fifth week
    D. sixth week   (8:98)

60. At the end of the fourth week of development, the embryo measures
    A. 2 mm
    B. 4 mm
    C. 5 mm
    D. 10 mm   (8:100)

61. At eight weeks, the embryo measures approximately
    A. 1.2 in.
    B. 2.2 in.
    C. 3 in.
    D. 4.8 in.   (8:101)

62. The sex of the embryo can first be determined at the
    A. eighth week
    B. tenth week
    C. twelfth week
    D. fourteenth week   (8:102)

63. The kidneys start secreting at what fetal age?
    A. twelfth week
    B. fourteenth week
    C. sixteenth week
    D. eighteenth week   (8:101)

64. At the twelfth week of fetal development the fetus weighs approximately
    A. 1 g
    B. 14 g
    C. 28 g
    D. 42 g   (8:102)

65. At the twelfth week of fetal development the fetus measures approximately
    A. 3 cm
    B. 7 cm
    C. 10 cm
    D. 14 cm   (8:102)

66. The fetus that weighs approximately 300 g is said to be at what age of gestation?
    A. 16 weeks
    B. 18 weeks
    C. 20 weeks
    D. 22 weeks   (8:102)

67. Vernix caseosa first appears on the skin of the fetus at about what week of gestation?
    A. sixteenth week
    B. eighteenth week
    C. twentieth week
    D. twenty-second week   (8:103)

68. The buds for the permanent teeth begin to develop at about what week of gestation?

    A. sixteenth week
    B. eighteenth week
    C. twentieth week
    D. twenty-second week   (8:102)

69. Fat deposits in the skin make their appearance at about what week of fetal life?

    A. twentieth week
    B. twenty-second week
    C. twenty-fourth week
    D. twenty-sixth week   (8:103)

70. At the end of the thirty-second week of gestation the fetus weighs approximately

    A. 1,500 g
    B. 1,700 g
    C. 2,000 g
    D. 2,500 g   (8:104)

71. Which of the following body systems is the first to appear in the embryo?

    A. circulatory system
    B. gastrointestinal system
    C. nervous system
    D. urinary system   (8:105)

72. The kidneys begin to secrete about what time in fetal life?

    A. fifth week
    B. seventh week
    C. ninth week
    D. none of the above   (8:105)

73. The fetus is capable of swallowing amniotic fluid at about what week of fetal life?

    A. tenth week
    B. sixteenth week
    C. twentieth week
    D. twenty-fourth week   (8:105)

74. Which of the following body systems is the last to mature?

    A. nervous system
    B. reproductive system
    C. respiratory system
    D. gastrointestinal system   (8:105)

75. Grasp reflex is present in the fetus by the

    A. second month
    B. third month
    C. fourth month
    D. fifth month   (8:105)

76. Movement in the unborn child starts about the

    A. second month
    B. third month
    C. fourth month
    D. fifth month   (8:105)

77. The term "viable" means

    A. subject to changes
    B. alive
    C. able or likely to live
    D. none of the above   (2:43)

78. A fetus measuring 15 cm in length and weighing 100 g probably has a gestational age of about

    A. 8 weeks
    B. 12 weeks
    C. 16 weeks
    D. 20 weeks   (8:102)

79. A fetus weighing about 1,100 g and measuring 35 cm in length probably has a gestational age of about

    A. 24 weeks
    B. 28 weeks
    C. 32 weeks
    D. 36 weeks   (8:103–4)

80. At what age of fetal life do the teeth begin to form?

    A. end of fifth week
    B. end of twelfth week
    C. end of sixteenth week
    D. end of twentieth week   (8:101)

81. At what age of fetal life do the external genitalia become evident?

    A. end of first lunar month
    B. end of second lunar month
    C. end of third lunar month
    D. end of fourth lunar month   (4:112)

82. At the end of the sixth lunar month the fetus has attained what percentage of its length?

    A. 40%
    B. 50%
    C. 60%
    D. 70%   (8:95)

83. The third phase of the fetal period occurs when the

    A. organs and systems are established
    B. organs and systems start functioning
    C. organs and systems develop to the stage

where they can function outside of the uterus
- D. organs and systems start functioning outside of the uterus (8:95)

84. Nucleated red blood cells are formed in which of the following structures during fetal life?
    1. yolk sac
    2. placenta
    3. liver
    4. spleen
    5. lymph tissue
    - A. 1, 2
    - B. 1, 3, 4
    - C. 3, 4, 5
    - D. all of the above (6:94)

85. Which of the following organs is responsible for the body temperature of the fetus?
    - A. amniotic fluid
    - B. placenta
    - C. mother's body temperature
    - D. control is within the fetus (6:82)

86. Closure of the foramen ovale is permanent by the end of the year in what percentage of all infants?
    - A. 100%
    - B. 75%
    - C. 50%
    - D. 25% (6:101)

87. Which of the following fetal structures provides for the passage of blood from an artery to an artery?
    - A. ductus arteriosus
    - B. hypogastric arteries
    - C. ductus venosus
    - D. umbilical arteries (6:99–101)

88. Which of the following fetal structures provides for the passage of blood from a vein to a vein?
    - A. ductus arteriosus
    - B. ductus venosus
    - C. foramen ovale
    - D. none of the above (6:99)

89. The hypogastric arteries
    - A. carry pure blood to the inferior vena cava
    - B. carry impure blood to the fetal liver
    - C. return impure blood to the placenta
    - D. carry pure blood from the placenta (6:101)

90. The purpose of the foramen ovale is to shunt the
    - A. oxygenated blood from the right into the left atrium
    - B. impure blood from the left to the right ventricle
    - C. oxygenated blood from the right atrium to the right ventricle
    - D. impure blood from the right atrium to the right ventricle (6:99)

91. Which of the following structures also assists in the transfer of the blood from the right to the left atrium during intrauterine life?
    - A. mitral valve
    - B. tricuspid valve
    - C. eustachian valve
    - D. fossa ovalis (6:99)

92. The ductus arteriosus is
    - A. a direct opening between the right and left atrium of the heart
    - B. a fetal vessel connecting the pulmonary artery and the aorta
    - C. a fetal blood vessel connecting the umbilical vein and the inferior vena cava
    - D. none of the above (8:106)

93. During intrauterine life, the umbilical vein
    - A. brings arterial blood to the liver and heart
    - B. shunts arterial blood into the inferior vena cava
    - C. transports arteriovenous blood to the placenta
    - D. receives blood from both ventricles (4:119)

94. Fetal circulation differs from adult circulation in which of the following ways?
    1. there is an opening between the right and left atrium
    2. there is a shunt between the pulmonary artery and the aorta
    3. there are necessary structures such as the umbilical cord
    4. there is a dextroposition of the aorta
    - A. 1
    - B. 1, 2
    - C. 1, 2, 3
    - D. 1, 2, 3, 4 (4:117–8)

95. Following formation of the chorion, the implanted blastocyst is called the
    - A. seminal vesicle

B. chorionic vesicle
C. secondary follicle
D. none of the above (8:84)

96. The chorion arises from what structure?

A. trophoblasts
B. embryoblast
C. ectoderm
D. mesoderm (8:84)

97. The first source of nutrition to the growing organism is

A. secretions from uterine glands
B. yolk sac
C. tails of the sperm
D. none of the above (8:86)

98. The organism first receives its outside nutrition via what structure?

A. trophoblasts
B. yolk sac
C. chorionic villi
D. none of the above (4:116)

99. The chorionic villi begin to form

A. immediately at conception
B. during the traveling time of the fertilized ovum
C. at implantation
D. about the end of the second week of life (8:85)

100. Which of the following functions is *not* attributed to the placenta?

A. internal organ of reproduction
B. endocrine organ
C. kidney organ for fetus
D. living organ for fetus (8:86)

101. Nutritive substances reach the embryonic cells by

A. osmosis
B. diffusion
C. cytolysis
D. none of the above (8:86)

102. A maternal circulation is formed by the end of the

A. first week of life
B. second week of life
C. third week of life
D. fourth week of life (8:87)

103. The placenta is formed from what fetal structure?

A. chorion villi
B. chorion frondosum

C. yolk sac
D. none of the above (8:87)

104. At what point during gestation are the weight of the placenta and the fetus equal?

A. before the fourth month
B. at the fourth month
C. at the sixth month
D. at term (8:87)

105. The reservoir that contains the pooled maternal blood is called the

A. lactiferous sinus
B. intervillous space
C. epididymal bodies
D. none of the above (8:87)

106. The above-mentioned reservoir of the placenta contains about how much blood?

A. 75 mL
B. 150 mL
C. 200 mL
D. 300 mL (8:87)

107. The rate of maternal blood circulating through the placenta has been estimated at

A. 100 to 200 mL/min
B. 500 to 600 mL/min
C. 50 to 100 mL/min
D. 700 to 800 mL/min (8:87)

108. The transfer of substances from mother to fetus and from fetus to mother takes place through the

A. endometrial arteries and veins
B. chorionic villi
C. umbilical veins
D. placental arteries (8:88)

109. Exchange of substances in the mature placental organ is accomplished by which of the following?

1. diffusion
2. osmosis
3. selective power of the villi cells
4. ability of villi cells to alter substances as necessary

A. 2
B. 1, 3, 4
C. 1
D. all of the above (6:84; 8:88)

110. The yolk sac ceases to grow

A. at conception
B. at about the first week of life

C. as soon as circulation is established between chorionic villi and embryonic vessels

D. at 12 weeks of gestation   (6:55)

111. At maturity, the placenta is about

A. 2 in. in diameter, 0.25 in. thick
B. 5 in. in diameter, 0.50 in. thick
C. 8 in. in diameter, 1 in. thick
D. 10 in. in diameter, 2 in. thick   (4:108)

112. The various segments of the placenta are called

A. septa
B. Duncan's bodies
C. subchorial cavities
D. cotyledons   (4:110)

113. At the fifth month of gestation the placenta covers approximately what percentage of the uterus?

A. 25%
B. 50%
C. 77%
D. 80%   (6:81)

114. Growth of the placenta ceases at about the

A. ninth month of gestation
B. onset of labor
C. eighth month of gestation
D. seventh month of gestation   (6:82)

115. The placenta is formed by the end of the

A. second month
B. third month
C. fourth month
D. first month   (4:110)

116. At the time of separation from the uterine wall at term, the placenta is

A. 2 to 4 in. in diameter, 0.50 in. thick at center
B. 6 to 8 in. in diameter, 0.50 in. thick at center
C. 6 to 8 in. in diameter, 1 in. thick at center
D. 10 in. in diameter, 2 in. thick at center   (8:90)

117. Which of the following are known to transfer from the placenta to the fetus?

1. chickenpox
2. diphtheria
3. rubella
4. toxoplasmosis
4. smallpox

A. 1, 2, 5
B. 3, 4
C. 1, 2, 3, 5
D. all of the above   (6:85)

118. Which of the following is associated with the placental dysfunction syndrome?

A. preeclampsia
B. excessive smoking
C. severe malnutrition
D. all of the above   (6:56)

119. What is the name of the two groups of cells that separate fetal from maternal blood flow?

1. Sertoli
2. syncytial
3. epithelial
4. Leydig
5. Langhans'

A. 1, 4
B. 3, 5
C. 2, 5
D. none of the above   (6:54)

120. The average amount of amniotic fluid at term is between

A. 8 and 16 oz
B. 16 and 32 oz
C. 24 and 48 oz
D. 36 and 72 oz   (8:83)

121. Which of the following substances is *not* normally found in amniotic fluid?

A. fetal urine
B. epithelial cells
C. flecks of fetal skin
D. all of the above   (8:83)

122. In reference to the source of amniotic fluid, which of the following reflects the most accepted concept?

A. it is a maternal transudate
B. it is secreted by cells in the amniotic fluid
C. it is produced by fetal lungs and kidneys
D. it is not definitely known   (8:83)

123. An amniocentesis for genetic analysis is usually performed between the

A. tenth and twelfth week
B. fourteenth and eighteenth week
C. twentieth and twenty-fourth week
D. none of the above   (6:80)

124. In which of the following cases is amniocentesis usually being recommended?

    1. either parent a balanced translocation carrier
    2. previous child with a chromosomal defect
    3. mother under 17 years of age
    4. mother over 40 years of age
    5. both parents carriers for a diagnosable metabolic defect

    A. 1, 2, 5
    B. 1, 2, 3
    C. 1, 2, 3, 5
    D. all of the above   (3:215)

125. The most frequent complication of amniocentesis is

    A. premature labor
    B. amnionitis
    C. bleeding from the placenta
    D. none of the above   (6:81)

126. Which fetal disease was the first to be diagnosed by examining amniotic fluid cells?

    A. cystic fibrosis
    B. Tay-Sachs
    C. adrenogenital syndrome
    D. Hunter's syndrome   (6:81)

127. Which of the following abnormalities can be diagnosed in utero?

    1. Niemann-Pick disease
    2. Tay-Sachs disease
    3. Lesch-Nuham disease
    4. glycogen storage disease
    5. galactosemia

    A. 2, 4, 5
    B. 1, 2, 3
    C. all of the above
    D. none of the above   (3:215)

128. Many of the common congenital abnormalities such as cleft lip, cleft palate, and pyloric stenosis are inherited in which one of the following ways?

    A. dominantly
    B. recessively
    C. sex-linked
    D. polygenically   (3:210)

129. Who described the first chromosomal abnormality?

    A. LeJeune
    B. Lynch

C. McKusick
D. none of the above   (3:217−8)

130. When were human chromosomes first accurately counted?

    A. 1932
    B. 1944
    C. 1956
    D. none of the above   (3:217)

131. Which of the following maternal age groups are most likely to have offspring with congenital abnormalities?

    1. 15- to 17-year age group
    2. 14- to 20-year age group
    3. 25- to 30-year age group
    4. 35- to 40-year age group

    A. 1, 2,
    B. 1, 4
    C. all of the above
    D. none of the above   (6:105)

132. Which of the following are considered to be clinical features of the child who has Down's syndrome?

    1. large head
    2. high palate
    3. harelip
    4. short broad hands
    5. curved fifth finger

    A. 1, 2, 3
    B. 2, 3, 5
    C. 2, 4, 5
    D. all of the above   (3:202)

133. Which of the following are considered to be clinical features of the child who has Turner's syndrome?

    1. short stature
    2. excessive nevi
    3. broad chest
    4. webbed neck
    5. low hairline

    A. 1, 3, 5
    B. 2
    C. 4, 5
    D. all of the above   (3:205)

134. Turner's syndrome is caused by

    A. an abnormal number of sex chromosomes
    B. an inborn error of metabolism
    C. an autosomal defect
    D. an acquired defect   (8:756)

135. The incidence of congenital abnormalities is estimated to be what percentage of all pregnancies?
    A. 1 to 3%
    B. 3 to 5%
    C. 5 to 8%
    D. 8 to 10%   (3:199)

136. Approximately what percentage of spontaneous abortions will show chromosomal aberration in the fetus?
    A. 5%
    B. 10%
    C. 15 to 25%
    D. 25 to 50%   (3:288)

137. The most common autosomal defect is that of
    A. Down's syndrome
    B. Turner's syndrome
    C. Klinefelter's syndrome
    D. phenylketonuria   (3:200)

138. Children with Down's syndrome are most commonly born to mothers in which age group?
    A. 15- to 20-year age group
    B. 20- to 25-year age group
    C. 35- to 40-year age group
    D. 40- to 45-year age group   (6:105)

139. The most common type of Down's syndrome born to the younger mother is that of
    A. translocation Down's syndrome
    B. trisomy 21
    C. mosaicism
    D. none of the above   (3:202–3)

140. Radiation exposure causes the *most* damage to the developing fetus at what period of fetal development?
    A. two to six weeks
    B. three to five months
    C. six to nine months
    D. all of the above   (3:816)

141. Midline anomalies such as spina bifida occulta, or meningocele, occur during what period of fetal development?
    A. by the end of the second week
    B. by the end of the fourth week
    C. by the end of the sixth week
    D. by the end of the eighth week   (3:817)

142. The cleft lip and/or cleft palate occur during what period of fetal development?
    A. between third and fifth weeks
    B. between fifth and eighth weeks
    C. between ninth and twelfth weeks
    D. between twelfth and sixteenth weeks   (3:820)

143. Tracheoesophageal fistula occurs during what period of fetal development?
    A. by the fourth week
    B. by the sixth week
    C. by the eighth week
    D. by the twelfth week   (3:822)

144. Imperforate anus occurs during what period of fetal development?
    A. by the sixth week
    B. by the eight week
    C. by the tenth week
    D. by the twelfth week   (3:823)

145. Omphalocele occurs during what period of fetal development?
    A. between the fifth and seventh week
    B. between the seventh and tenth week
    C. between the tenth and thirteenth week
    D. none of the above   (3:823)

146. Congenital dislocation of the hip occurs during what period of fetal development?
    A. seventh embryonic week
    B. ninth embryonic week
    C. eleventh embryonic week
    D. thirteenth embryonic week   (3:829)

147. Transposition of the great vessels is characterized by a condition in which
    A. there is a small right ventricle and a small tricuspid valve
    B. the aorta arises from the right ventricle, and the pulmonary arteries arise from the left ventricle
    C. the aorta arises from the left ventricle, and the pulmonary arteries arise from the right ventricle
    D. there is pulmonary stenosis, a ventricular septal defect, dextroposition of the aorta, and the right ventricular hypertrophy   (3:827)

148. Approximately what percentage of malformations in the newborn can be attributed to known causes?
    A. 1%

B. 10%
C. 15%
D. 25%   (3:813)

149. Which organism has been known to cause hydrocephalus, microcephalus, cerebral dysfunctions, and visceral and skeletal malformation?

A. cytomegalovirus
B. rubella virus
C. coxsackievirus
D. *Treponema pallidum*   (3:814)

150. A folic acid deficiency in the mother can result in which of the following abnormalities in the newborn?

A. club feet
B. anencephaly
C. absence of fetal limbs
D. none of these   (6:106)

151. Current research indicates that a toxin or drug of what molecular weight can cross the placenta?

A. 250
B. 350
C. 800
D. all of these   (6:108)

152. Which of the following men observed a definite relationship between congenital cataracts and maternal rubella?

A. M. Fishbein
B. N. McAlister Gregg
C. F. Hecht
D. none of the above   (6:108)

153. Which of the following men in 1966 developed a live, attenuated rubella virus vaccine?

1. Louis Bourgeois
2. Harry Meyer
3. Paul Parkman
4. John William Ballantyne

A. 1, 3
B. 2, 3
C. 2, 4
D. none of the above   (6:108)

154. When is the best time to administer attenuated rubella virus vaccine?

A. first trimester of pregnancy
B. second trimester of pregnancy
C. third trimester of pregnancy
D. postpartum period   (6:109)

155. If a woman contracts rubella during her third trimester of pregnancy the child will

A. have congenital abnormalities
B. not be affected
C. have a mild case of rubella that lasts for about six weeks following birth
D. secrete the rubella virus in his urine for about a year following birth   (6:108)

156. If a mother contracts smallpox during pregnancy what are the chances that she will abort the fetus?

A. 5%
B. 10%
C. 50%
D. none of the above   (6:110)

157. Which of the following theories have been advanced regarding the transmission of syphilis to the fetus?

A. Langhans' layer of chorion forms a barrier that prevents the passage of the *Treponema pallidum* prior to the sixteenth week of gestation
B. fetus swallows the amniotic fluid that contains the spirochetes prior to the sixteenth week of gestation
C. both A and B
D. neither A nor B   (4:594)

158. Which of the following drugs have been found useful in treating syphilis?

A. penicillin
B. cephaloridine
C. erythromycin
D. all of the above   (6:110)

159. Which of the following fetal disorders may be treated during intrauterine life?

1. Tay-Sachs disease
2. erythroblastosis fetalis
3. maple syrup urine disease
4. adrenogenital syndrome
5. Hunter's syndrome

A. 1, 2
B. 2, 3
C. 2, 4
D. none of the above   (6:104,118)

160. At what age is the fetus able to open and close its eyes?

A. end of fourth lunar month
B. end of fifth lunar month
C. end of sixth lunar month
D. end of seventh lunar month   (2:86)

161. Who is given credit for performing the first successful intrauterine transfusion?

    A. Dr. David Hawkins
    B. Dr. Brian Little
    C. Dr. William Lily
    D. none of the above   (6:118)

162. Erythroblastosis occurs

    A. once in every 200 pregnancies
    B. once in every 250 pregnancies
    C. once in every 300 pregnancies
    D. none of the above   (6:117)

163. What is the name of the test used to determine whether vaginal bleeding is from a maternal or fetal source?

    A. Coombs' test
    B. Downey-Apt test
    C. Farber's test
    D. none of the above   (6:192)

164. Approximately how long does it take for the spermatozoa to mature?

    A. 20 days
    B. 44 days
    C. 64 days
    D. 72 days   (8:64)

165. The term used to define fertilization of two ova from two sperm from different males occurring at about the same time is

    A. superfecundation
    B. superfetation
    C. fornication
    D. none of the above   (4:688)

166. When the umbilical cord is attached along the margin of the placenta, the condition is termed

    A. placenta circumvallata
    B. placenta succenturiata
    C. placenta battledore
    D. none of the above   (6:85)

167. The name given to the segregation of tissues into various organs during embryonic development is

    A. mitosis
    B. organogenesis
    C. gametogenesis
    D. none of the above   (6:106)

168. It has been estimated that twins occur

    A. once in 70 pregnancies
    B. once in 90 pregnancies
    C. once in 100 pregnancies
    D. once in 150 pregnancies   (8:193)

169. Triplets occur once in every

    A. 600 births
    B. 1,000 births
    C. 6,000 births
    D. 9,000 births   (8:93)

170. Who of the following is *most* likely to have twins?

    A. adolescent with her first pregnancy
    B. older woman with her first pregnancy
    C. adolescent with her second pregnancy
    D. older woman with her third pregnancy   (2:185)

171. Following maturation the male and female germ cells are called

    A. gametes
    B. zygotes
    C. morulas
    D. none of the above   (8:66)

172. How long does it take the sperm to reach the ovum?

    A. several minutes
    B. several hours
    C. less than 24 hours
    D. more than 24 hours   (8:76)

173. The series of rapid mitotic divisions that results in the cells that are termed blastomeres is termed

    A. gastrulation
    B. gametogenesis
    C. cleavage
    D. none of the above   (8:79)

174. During the process of placental transfer, some substances are actually engulfed by the fetal cells. The term used to describe this process is

    A. dialysis
    B. osmosis
    C. pinocytosis
    D. cytolysis   (6:84)

175. The diameter of the ovum is approximately

    A. 0.01 mm
    B. 0.1 mm
    C. 0.2 mm
    D. 0.4 mm   (8:75)

176. At the time of implantation, the diameter of the developing organism is approximately
   A. 1/10 in.
   B. 1/100 in.
   C. 1/200 in.
   D. 1/250 in.   (8:80)

177. The term "placenta" comes from a Latin word meaning
   A. sieve
   B. cake
   C. reservoir
   D. the term does not come from a Latin word   (4:110)

178. The sex of the unborn child can be detected by which of the following methods?
   A. examination of the sex chromatin pattern in the cells that float in the amniotic fluid
   B. ultrasound testing during the last 10 weeks of pregnancy
   C. measuring the level of testosterone in the maternal urine between the sixth and tenth week of gestation
   D. all of the above   (6:86—7)

179. When doing chromosomal studies, which of the following substances can be added to blood samples to stimulate mitosis?
   A. aceto-orcein
   B. phytohemagglutinin
   C. griseofulvin
   D. Ilosone   (3:199)

180. Chromosomal studies of the individual cells are done during which phase of cell division?
   A. metaphase
   B. anaphase
   C. telophase
   D. prophase   (4:96)

181. The drug used to arrest cell division during chromosomal counts is
   A. colchicine
   B. feulgen
   C. Nesacaine
   D. none of the above   (3:199)

182. During fetal life the umbilical cord
   A. floats in the amniotic fluid in a lifeless manner
   B. is pressed close to the fetus because of the pressure within the uterus
   C. tends to be stiff and inflexible because of the force of the blood flowing through it
   D. can encircle the neck of the fetus as a result of "stretching motions" on the part of the mother   (5:47)

183. Approximately how long is the spermatozoan?
   A. 0.06 mm
   B. 0.02 mm
   C. 0.1 mm
   D. none of the above   (8:74)

Directions: Each group of numbered words or phrases is followed by a list of lettered statements. MATCH the lettered statement with the numbered word or phrase most closely associated with it.

Questions 184 through 187
184. membrane that forms outside the boundary of the cytoplasm before fertilization
185. term used to describe the sperm after separation of its head from the rest of the body before fertilization
186. membrane that surrounds the ovum before fertilization
187. term used to describe the cells that adhere to the ovum's outer surfaces before fertilization
   A. vitelline membrane
   B. pronucleus
   C. corona radiata
   D. zona pellucida   (8:73—6)

Questions 188 through 191
188. cells that form the middle germ layer of the embedded ovum
189. cells that form the outer germ layer of the embedded ovum
190. uterine lining that lies directly beneath the embedded ovum
191. uterine lining which is pushed out by the embedded ovum
   A. ectoderm
   B. decidua capsularis
   C. mesoderm
   D. decidua basalis   (2:54)

Questions 192 through 195
192. portion of the trophoblasts that comes in contact with the decidua basalis
193. portion of the trophoblasts that comes in contact with the decidua vera
194. structure formed by the union of the chorionic villi and the decidua basalis

195. forerunner of the umbilical cord

    A. body stalk
    B. placenta
    C. chorion frondosum
    D. chorion laeve   (6:77)

Questions 196 through 199

196. observation of the color of the amniotic fluid
197. visualization of fetus and placenta
198. measurement of fetal biparietal diameters
199. analysis of amniotic fluid

    A. amniocentesis
    B. amnioscopy
    C. diagnostic ultrasound
    D. amniography   (6:101−3)

Questions 200 through 203

200. endometrium
201. ectoderm
202. endoderm
203. amnion

    A. internal layer of fetal membranes
    B. innermost layer of the primitive embryo
    C. innermost mucous layer of the uterus
    D. outer layers of cells of the primitive embryo   (2:54,69−70)

Questions 204 through 207

204. nail beds form on fingers and toes
205. pulsation starts
206. blood vessels are visible beneath the skin
207. the nerves develop

    A. first to fourth week
    B. sixth to eighth week
    C. ninth to twelfth week
    D. thirteenth to sixteenth week   (6:92)

Questions 208 through 211

208. membrane disappears from eyes and eyelids reopen
209. testicles may be in scrotal sac
210. fetal thyroid begins to function
211. fingernails and toenails can be distinguished

    A. thirteenth to fifteenth week
    B. seventeenth to twentieth week
    C. twenty-fifth to twenty-eighth week
    D. twenty-ninth to thirty-second week
                                                (6:90−1)

Questions 212 through 215

212. dicumarol
213. cortisone
214. analgesics
215. sulfonamides

    A. kernicterus
    B. reduced thermal stability of newborn
    C. hemorrhage, fetal death
    D. lip and palate deformities   (6:112)

Answers and Explanations:
Physiology and Development of the Fetus

1. **D.** All body cells in an organism have an identical number of chromosomes that is characteristic for the organism in which they exist.

2. **C.** Each cell contains 22 pairs of autosomes and one pair of sex chromosomes.

3. **B.** In all human cells with the exception of the mature sex cells there are normally 46 chromosomes. However, prior to fertilization each gamete undergoes a reduction in its total number of chromosomes to half the usual number.

4. **A.** Male cells normally contain one X and one Y chromosome.

5. **C.** The chromosomes are placed in seven groups according to length, size, and position of the centromere.

6. **A.** The sex chromosomes are designed as XX in the female cell and XY in the male cell.

7. **A.** The nucleus of the sperm contains 23 chromosomes.

8. **B.** When the sperm enters the ovum, the head detaches from the body. The remaining cell is called the male pronucleus. The ovum completes its maturation by separation of the second polar body. The chromosomes that remain organize themselves into a nucleus called the female pronucleus. The fertilized ovum is now a zygote with 46 chromosomes.

9. **B.** Prior to fertilization, the number of chromosomes is reduced by half during the process of meiosis.

10. **B.** A chromosome is a dark-staining, rod-shaped body.

11. **B.** Genotype is a description of the genetic makeup of an individual with respect to a given characteristic.

12. **B.** The process of meiosis matures the ovum and prepares the chromosomes for fertilization.

13. **B.** The ovum is suspended in a fluid that is called cytoplasm.

14. **B.** The deposit of the sperm into the vagina is called semination.

15. **D.** All of the terms mentioned mean fertilization or fusion of the male and female pronuclei.

16. **B.** The sperm releases the enzyme hyaluronidase, which acts on the zona pellucida —the protective covering surrounding the ovum. This makes penetration possible.

17. **D.** The ovum has a life of 24 hours or less.

18. **C.** The sperm has a fertilizing capacity for no more than 48 hours.

19. **C.** At each ejaculation, the climax of intercourse in the male, about 300 million sperm are discharged into the vagina.

20. **D.** Fertilization usually occurs in the distal end of the fallopian tube.

21. **C.** The developing embryo is propelled by both the ciliary current and the muscular contractions within the tube.

22. **B.** At this time the single cell begins to develop as an embryo.

23. **B.** Approximately 33% of all twins are of the identical type.

24. **D.** Fertilization of one ovum may result in a single male or female child pregnancy and monozygotic or identical twins.

25. **D.** Triplets may derive from one ovum, as in the case of twins, or from two or three ova. Accordingly, there may be single-, double-, or triple-ovum triplets.

26. **C.** The early cell divisions produce a solid ball of cells called the morula.

27. **B.** It takes the fertilized ovum six to seven days to travel to the uterus, and it is fully implanted in the uterine wall by the end of fourteen days.

28. **C.** The ovum is in the blastocyst stage at the time of implantation.

29. **B.** This is the period when the lining of the uterus has reached its greatest thickness.

30. **B.** If pregnancy occurs, the already thickened endometrium becomes even thicker, the cells enlarge, and the structure becomes known as the decidua.

31. **B.** The trophoblastic cells, the outer covering of the blastocyst, secrete proteolytic and cytolytic enzymes, which assist them in burrowing their way into the compact layer of the endometrium.

32. **C.** Implantation of the fertilized ovum occurs approximately seven days after conception.

33. **B.** The decidua reaches its maximum height, about 10 mm, at the third or fourth month of pregnancy, after which it begins to thin until it is 1 to 2 mm thick at the end of the pregnancy.

34. **C.** When this hormone was first extracted from the placenta it was called human placental lactogen because of its effect on lactational changes in mammary tissue. Later it was discovered that this same hormone produced growth-like effects, and it was renamed chorionic growth hormone prolactin. In 1968 it was again called human chorionic somatomammotropin.

35. **B.** The syncytial cells (of the trophoblasts) produce progesterone.

36. **B.** Chorionic gonadotropin stimulates the corpus luteum to be continued.

37. **B.** Chorionic gonadotropin is the hormone that provides the basis for the pregnancy tests.

38. **D.** Interstitial cell-stimulating hormone is not produced by the placenta.

39. **B.** The amnion is the inner of the two fetal membranes and comes in direct contact with the amniotic fluid.

40. **D.** All of the factors mentioned are considered to be important functions. All appear to be directed toward maintaining an optimal environment for the fetus during intrauterine development.

41. **D.** The fetus begins to swallow amniotic fluid by the fourth month of development, and by the time it reaches full term it swallows as much as 450 mL/day.

42. **A.** At the end of the sixth month there is approximately 1,000 to 1,500 mL of amniotic fluid. The amount then begins to decrease.

43. **B.** The pH of amniotic fluid is slightly alkaline, pH 7.2.

44. **C.** About 35% of the amniotic fluid is replaced every hour.

45. **B.** The entoderm is the inner germ layer. The following structures develop from the entoderm: the alimentary canal, the thymus, thyroid, liver, lungs, pancreas, bladder, and the various small glands and tubules.

46. **A.** From conception till about the eighth week of pregnancy the developing organism is called the embryo.

47. **C.** The body stalk is the forerunner of the umbilical cord.

48. **B.** At term, the umbilical cord measures about 55 cm (22 in.), but it may vary from 30 to 100 cm (12 to 39 in.).

49. **B.** It has been shown that one of the naturally occurring prostaglandins is present in Wharton's jelly. Researchers believe that the vasoconstrictive effect of this prostaglandin inhibits bleeding from the umbilical cord stump.

50. **B.** The umbilical cord contains two arteries and one vein and is covered by Wharton's jelly.

51. **B.** In the fetus the oxygenated blood flows up the cord through the umbilical vein.

52. **B.** Approximately half a pint of blood flows through the umbilical cord every minute.

53. **B.** Haase's rule is as follows: Take the square root of the length of the fetus in centimeters for the first five months and after this, multiply the length of the fetus by five.

54. **B.** And the average length of pregnancy from the first day of the last menstrual period is 280 days.

55. **B.** The level of creatinine in the amniotic fluid increases with gestational age. A level of 2 mg/dL is to be expected of a gestational age of 37 weeks.

56. **B.** Growth and development always occur in the upper parts of the body first and then in the lower parts. This is known as cephalocaudal development.

57. **C.** The exact time of fertilization cannot be known. Therefore, the age of the embryo can be known with a certain amount of certainty if one counts from the fourteenth day after the onset of the last menstrual period.

58. **C.** By the end of the fourth week the majority of the body systems have begun to appear in rudimentary form.

59. **B.** By the end of the first month the fetal heart is beating, and there is an established blood flow.

60. **C.** At the end of the fourth week of development, the embryo measures about 5 mm (0.2 in.).

61. **A.** At eight weeks of age the embryo measures approximately 1.2 in. from crown to heel.

62. **C.** The sex of the fetus can be determined by the end of the twelfth week.

63. **A.** The kidneys are capable of secreting early in the third month.

64. **B.** At the end of the twelfth week the fetus weighs approximately 14 g (a half oz).

65. **B.** At the end of the twelfth week of development the fetus is about 7 cm (2.9 in.) long from crown to heel.

66. **C.** By the end of the twentieth week the fetus weighs approximately 300 g (11 oz).

67. **C.** Vernix caseosa, a substance consisting of secretion from the sebaceous glands, appears on the skin of the fetus at the end of the twentieth week.

68. **C.** By the twentieth week the buds for the permanent teeth have begun to develop.

69. **C.** By the end of the twenty-fourth week there is a beginning deposit of fat beneath the skin.

70 **B.** At the end of the thirty-second week of development the fetus weighs approximately 1,700 g (3 lb, 12 oz).

71. **C.** The nervous system is the first system to appear in the fetus. This may be evidenced by some movements and reflex activities at the end of the second month.

72. **C.** Secretion of the kidneys starts the ninth week of fetal life.

73. **B.** The fetus begins to swallow amniotic fluid at about the sixteenth week of development.

74. **B.** The reproductive system is the last body system to mature.

75. **B.** The grasp reflex is present in the fetus by the third month.

76. **A.** Movements and reflex activities can be observed by the end of the second month of development in the fetus. However, the woman does not feel these movements for some time.

77. **C.** The ability of the fetus to sustain life outside the uterus usually develops between the twentieth and twenty-eighth week of gestation.

78. **C.** There is also lanugo on the body of the fetus, and there is meconium in the intestines.

79. **B.** The child appears thin, the skin reddish and covered with vernix. If born at the twenty-eighth week of gestation, the child's organs are sufficiently developed to make his chances for survival not entirely unfavorable.

80. **B.** The teeth are forming under the gums by the end of the twelfth week.

81. **B.** The external genitalia become evident by the end of the second lunar month, but at this time it is difficult to distinguish the sex of the child.

82. **C.** At the end of the sixth lunar month the fetus has attained about 60% of its length.

83. **C.** The third phase of the fetal period occurs when the fetal organs and systems develop to the stage where they can function in extrauterine life.

84. **D.** The nucleated red blood cells are formed in all the structures mentioned. The formation of the cells takes place first in the yolk sac. Following this, they form in the placenta at about the third week of development. The liver begins to form cells at about six weeks, and by the twelfth week the spleen and lymph tissue also are producing the red blood cells.

85. **B.** The placenta regulates the body temperature of the fetus, which is 0.5°F warmer than the mother's.

86. **C.** Closure of the foramen ovale is permanent by the end of the first year in about 50% of all infants.

87. **A.** The ductus arteriosus is the vessel that carries blood from the pulmonary artery to the descending arch of the aorta.

88. **B.** The doctus venosus is the vessel that carries oxygenated blood from the umbilical vein to the inferior vena cava.

89. **C.** The hypogastric arteries branch off from the internal iliac arteries and are known as the umbilical arteries when they enter the umbilical cord.

90. **A.** The foramen ovale is an opening between the right and left atria.

91. **C.** The eustachian valve is a small structure in the foramen ovale.

92. **B.** The ductus anteriosus is a fetal vessel connecting the pulmonary artery and the aorta.

93. **A.** During uterine life the umbilical vein brings arterial blood to the liver and heart.

94. **C.** The opening between the right and left atrium is the foramen ovale. The shunt between the pulmonary artery and the aorta is the ductus arteriosus. The umbilical cord is present and functioning only during intrauterine life.

95. **B.** At this time the blastocyst is called a chorionic vesicle and is surrounded by a "lake" of maternal blood that has been created during implantation.

96. **A.** The chorion arises from the trophoblasts in the area devoid of the chorionic villi.

97. **B.** The yolk sac is a single layer of entodermal and mesodermal cells that are filled with albuminous material.

98. **A.** Before the chorionic villi begin to form (during the second week of embryonic development), the trophoblasts serve as a membrane through which nutritive materials reach the organism.

99. **D.** Villi begin to form over the chorion during the second week of embryonic development.

100. **A.** The placenta is considered to be an accessory structure rather than an internal organ of reproduction.

101. **B.** Nutritive substances reach the embryonic cells by diffusion.

102. **B.** Maternal circulation is established in a period of slightly over two weeks.

103. **B.** The placenta is formed from the chorionic villi lying over the decidua basalis—that of the chorion frondosum. It is also to a small degree maternal in origin.

104. **B.** Prior to the fourth month, the placenta is heavier than the fetus, and at full term the weight of the placenta is about one-seventh that of the fetus.

105. **B.** The intervillous space of the placenta contains the maternal blood.

106. **B.** It has been estimated that the intervillous space can hold about 150 mL of blood.

107. **B.** The rate of blood flow through the placenta has been estimated to be about 500 to 600 mL/min.

108. **B.** The transfer of substances from mother to fetus and from fetus to mother takes place through the chorionic villi.

109. **B.** The exchange of substances in the mature placenta takes place by diffusion, selective powers of the villi cells, and by the ability of these cells to alter substances as necessary.

110. **C.** The yolk sac ceases to grow as soon as circulation is established between the chorionic villi and the embryonic vessels.

111. **C.** At maturity the placenta is about 8 in. in diameter and 1 in. thick.

112. **D.** The various segments of the mature placenta are termed cotyledons.

113. **B.** At the fifth month of gestation the placenta covers approximately 50% of the uterus.

114. **D.** The growth of the placenta ceases at about the seventh month of gestation.

115. **B.** The placenta has formed by about the third month.

116. **C.** At term, the placenta is 6 to 8 in. in diameter and is about 1 in. thick at the center.

117. **D.** All of the conditions mentioned can transfer from the placenta to the fetus.

118. **D.** All of the conditions mentioned are associated with placental dysfunction syndrome.

119. **C.** The syncytial and Langhans' cells function as semipermeable membranes and separate fetal from maternal blood flow.

120. **B.** The amount of amniotic fliud at term is between 16 and 32 oz.

121. **D.** All of the mentioned substances are normally found in the amniotic fluid.

122. **D.** The source of amniotic fluid is not definitely known.

123. **B.** An amniocentesis for genetic analysis is usually performed between the fourteenth and eighteenth week of gestation. At this time enough fluid is available for a sample to be obtained.

124. **C.** Although most genetic centers are recommending that anmiocentesis be done on all cases mentioned, there is some controversy regarding this procedure for the mother over 40 years of ago.

125. **C.** The most frequent complication of an amniocentesis is bleeding from the placenta. This bleeding may lead to increased sensitization of Rh negative mothers when the blood from the placenta enters the maternal blodstream.

126. **C.** The adrenogenital syndrome was the first disease to be diagnosed by examining amniotic fluid cells.

127. **C.** All of the abnormalities mentioned can be diagnosed in utero.

128. **D.** It is believed that in polygenic inheritance multiple genes contribute to these defects and that each individual has a threshold above which the abnormality will be manifest. The more severe the defect, the more predisposing the genes present.

129. **A.** Jerome LeJeune in 1959 first described the trisomy 21 associated with Down's syndrome.

130. **C.** Human chromosomes were first accurately counted in 1956 by J.H. Tjio and Albert Levan and by Charles Lord and John Hamerton. Prior to 1956 the chromosomal number was believed to be 48 rather than 46.

131. **B.** Studies have indicated that very young parents (15- to 17-year age group) and parents nearing the end of the reproductive phase (late 40s) are more likely to have offspring with congenital abnormalities.

132. **C.** The child with Down's syndrome, in addition to high palate, short broad hands, and curved fifth finger, may also have, among other features, small head, protrusion of the tongue, and short broad neck.

133. **D.** The child with Turner's syndrome may also have lymphedema, cubitus valgus, hyperconvex and/or deep-set nails, renal anomalies, and widely spaced hypoplastic nipples.

134. **A.** Turner's syndrome is caused by an abnormal number of sex chromosomes. One having the disease may have rudimentary ovaries and fail to develop full female characteristics.

135. **B.** The incidence of congenital abnormalities is estimated to be 3 to 5% of all births. This incidence may even be higher if an individual is followed into adulthood.

136. **D.** Up to 25 to 50% of spontaneous abortions will have a chromosomal aberration.

137. **A.** Down's syndrome is the most common autosomal defect.

138. **D.** The incidence of Down's syndrome in women between 40 and 45 is 1 in 45 births; in women between 20 and 25, the incidence is 1 in 2,500 births.

139. **B.** Trisomy 21 is the most common type of Down's syndrome born to a young woman.

140. **A.** Exposure to radiation can cause damage to the fetus at any period of the pregnancy. However, exposure during the second to sixth week of gestation is probably the most damaging.

141. **B.** The closure of the neutral tube is completed in the embryo by the fourth week of development. Therefore, the midline anomalies occur at this time.

142. **C.** The palatal processes fuse about one month after the fusion of maxillary or premaxillary processes, which occurs between the fifth and eighth weeks. Incomplete fusion of the palatal processes results in cleft lip or cleft palate or both.

143. **C.** At the fourth week of gestation there is development of the laryngotracheal groove into the larynx, trachea, and primordial lung tissue. By the eighth week the esophageal lumen is formed. Anomalies can occur if these processes are not completed correctly.

144. **C.** The differentiation of tissue and the separation into two systems, that of the rectum and the bladder, occurs by the eighth week. At this time any interference with the development of the anal-rectal structures may result in anomalies.

145. **B.** The persistence of the embryonic stage between the seventh and tenth week of fetal life has resulted in varying amounts of abdominal viscera lying within the umbilical cord.

146. **A.** The hip joint should develop from mesoderm at about the seventh week. However, at birth the fetal cartilaginous state persists.

147. **B.** Transposition of the great vessels is incompatible with life unless the foramen ovale or ductus arteriosus remains open or there is an intraventricular or intra-atrial septal defect.

148. **B.** At this time about 9% of fetal malformations can be attributed to gross chromosomal abnormalities and about 1% can be attributed to specific teratogenic agents.

149. **A.** Cytomegalovirus is a virus that is associated with chronic infections in human beings. This virus crosses the placental barrier during an unknown period during the pregnancy and initiates a chronic infection in the developing fetus.

150. **B.** Folic acid is necessary for human cell formation and tissue growth. Defects resulting from folic acid deficiency usually involve errors in fusion.

151. **D.** Many scientists believe that any toxin or drug with a molecular weight of less than 1,000 can cross the placenta.

152. **B.** Following a major epidemic of German measles in 1940, Dr. N. McAlister Gregg observed a definite relationship between congenital cataracts and maternal rubella.

153. **B.** Harry Meyer and Paul Parkman in April of 1966 announced the development of a live, attenuated rubella virus vaccine.

154. **D.** The best time to administer rubella attenuated virus is during the postpartum period. The attenuated virus has been known to cross the placental barrier during pregnancy. It has also been shown that an individual can become reinfected after vaccination and transmit the virus to a susceptible person, i.e., the fetus.

155. **D.** During the third trimester of pregnancy, the infant born of a mother who contracts rubella can also contract rubella but will not be malformed. However, the infant will secrete the virus in his urine for about a year and thus expose others to the disease.

156. **C.** Smallpox, when transferred to the fetus, will result in abortion in about 50% of all cases.

157. **A.** Syphilis is transmitted to the fetus after the sixteenth week of gestation. Thus it is believed that the spirochetes pass through the placenta after the Langhans' layer disappears at about the eighteenth week.

158. **D.** All of the drugs mentioned have been found useful in treating syphilis. Penicillin, however, is the most effective drug.

159. **C.** Erythroblastosis fetalis may be treated by intrauterine transfusions of O-Rh negative packed red cells. Adrenogenital syndrome has been treated by injections of cortisone directly into the fetus.

160. **C.** The fetus is able to open and close its eyes by the end of the sixth lunar month.

161. **C.** Dr. William Lily of New Zealand is given credit for performing the first successful intrauterine transfusion.

162. **A.** Erythroblastosis occurs once in every 200 pregnancies.

163. **B.** Bleeding from the vagina during pregnancy that does not affect the woman's vital signs may be of fetal origin. The Downey-Apt test is then done to determine the origin of the bleeding.

164. **C.** It takes about 64 days for the spermatozoa to mature.

165. **A.** However, the term superfetation means the impregnation of an ovum during the time of a pre-existing pregnancy.

166. **C.** A placenta battledore is one in which the umbilical cord is attached along the margin instead of centrally as in most placentas.

167. **B.** During organogenesis, the various organ primordia appear. This gradually merges into periods of growth and differentiation.

168. **B.** It has been estimated that twins occur once in every 90 pregnancies.

169. **D.** It has been estimated that triplets occur once in every 9,000 births.

170. **D.** Studies have indicated that if a woman is of higher parity and older her chances of having twins are greater.

171. **A.** The mature male and female germ cells are called gametes.

172. **B.** Under optimum conditions the sperm can reach the ovum within a very few hours.

173. **C.** The collection of cells that are formed as a result of the cleavage arrange themselves into the form of a hollow sphere, which is the blastula. Thus the blastocyst is formed.

174. **C.** Pinocytosis is the term given to the process by which some particles are transferred by being engulfed by the cells.

175. **C.** The actual diameter of the human ovum is approximately 0.2 mm.

176. **B.** At the time of implantation, the blastocyst is about 1/100 in. in diameter.

177. **B.** The mature placenta resembles a cake.

178. **D.** All of the tests mentioned can be used to determine the sex of the unborn child.

179. **B.** When added to peripheral blood, phytohemagglutinin will stimulate mitosis and agglutinate white blood cells.

180. **A.** During the metaphase the individual chromosomes are separated from one another.

181. **A.** The drug colchicine added to the culture medium causes arrest of the cells in the metaphase.

182. **C.** Thus, if fetal movement causes the cord to loop, the loops do not become tightly knotted.

183. **A.** The spermatozoan measures about 0.06 mm in length.

184. **A.** The ovum contains a relatively large amount of cytoplasm. The vitelline membrane forms the outside boundary of the cytoplasm.

185. **B.** After the sperm penetrates the ovum, the head of the sperm separates from the body, increases in size, and takes on the appearance of a typical nucleus. The sperm is now termed the male pronucleus.

186. **D.** The zona pellucida is a thick, tough membrane that surrounds the ovum.

187. **C.** The follicle cells that adhere to the ovum following discharge from the graafian follicle are termed corona radiata.

188. **C.** The mesoderm is the middle layer of the three germ layers.

189. **A.** The ectoderm is the outer covering layer of the three germ layers.

190. **D.** The decidua basalis lies directly under the developing ovum.

191. **B.** The decidua capsularis is pushed out by the developing ovum.

192. **C.** The chorion frondosum is the portion of the trophoblasts that comes in contact with the decidua basalis.

193. **D.** The chorion laeve is the portion of the trophoblasts that comes in contact with the decidua vera.

194. **B.** The placenta is the structure formed by the union of the chorionic villi and the decidua basalis.

195. **A.** The body stalk is the forerunner of the umbilical cord.

196. **B.** The doctor is able to observe the color of the amniotic fluid through the intact membrane with the use of amnioscopy.

197. **D.** The doctor is able to see the fetus and placenta with the use of amniography.

198. **C.** The doctor is able to measure the biparietal diameter of the fetus with the use of diagnostic ultrasound.

199. **A.** The doctor is able to analyze the amniotic fluid with amniocentesis.

200. **C.** The innermost mucous layer of the uterus is called the endometrium.

201. **D.** The outer layer of cells of the primitive embryo is called ectoderm.

202. **B.** The innermost layer of cells of the primitive embryo is called endoderm.

203. **A.** The internal layer of fetal membranes is called amnion.

204. **C.** The nail beds form on the fingers and toes between the ninth and twelfth week.

205. **A.** Pulsation starts between the first and fourth week, more exactly on about the twenty-fourth day.

206. **D.** Blood vessels are visible beneath the transparent skin between the thirteenth and sixteenth week.

207. **B.** The nerves develop during the fifth to eighth week.

208. **C.** The membrane disappears from the eyes and eyelids reopen during the twenty-fifth to twenty-eighth week of development.

209. **D.** During the twenty-ninth to thirty-second week, the testicles may be in the scrotal sac.

210. **A.** The fetal thyroid begins to function between the thirteenth and fifteenth week.

211. **B.** The fingernails and toenails can be distinguished between the seventeenth and twentieth week.

212. **C.** Dicumarol may produce fetal hemorrhage or death.

213. **D.** Cortisone may produce lip and palate deformities in the fetus.

214. **B.** Analgesics may produce reduced thermal stability of the newborn.

215. **A.** Sulfonamides may produce kernicterus in the fetus.

CHAPTER 4

Antepartal Period

During the antepartal period the nurse is in the unique position of being able to support and provide instruction to the pregnant woman and her husband.

In this chapter you will find questions on medical problems and nursing care as related to the antepartal period. Included are both the normal and abnormal aspects of the topics under consideration.

At the end of this chapter you will find a series of situational questions in which you will be asked to apply your knowledge and understanding of antepartal nursing.

The role of the nurse during the antepartal period is an ever-expanding one, and the knowledge it requires has great practical application outside of the hospital as well.

Directions: Each of the questions or incomplete statements below is followed by four suggested answers or completions. Select the BEST answer in each case.

1. Amenorrhea is usually present in the pregnant woman because of
   A. high levels of estrogen and low levels of progesterone
   B. high levels of progesterone and low levels of estrogen
   C. low levels of estrogen and progesterone
   D. high levels of estrogen and progesterone (3:282)

2. Which of the following hormones are produced during pregnancy?
   A. chorionic gonadotropin
   B. estrogen
   C. progesterone
   D. all of the above (8:121)

3. Changes that prepare the breasts for lactation are the result of
   A. ovarian hormones
   B. placental hormones
   C. anterior pituitary hormones
   D. all of the above (8:117)

4. The substance responsible for positive reactions to the A-Z and other similar pregnancy tests is
   A. estrogen
   B. prolactin
   C. chorionic gonadotropin
   D. relaxin (8:89)

5. Diagnosis of a pregnancy by means of urine tests can first be possible
   A. immediately after conception
   B. about one week after conception or three weeks after last menstrual period
   C. about two weeks after conception or four weeks after last menstrual period
   D. about three weeks after conception or five weeks after last menstrual period (8:89)

6. Which of the following statements best describes the status of the corpus luteum at about the twelfth week of pregnancy?
   A. secreting progesterone at high levels
   B. secreting estrogen at high levels
   C. secreting both estrogen and progesterone at high levels
   D. undergoing retrogressive changes with decreased secretory activity (8:34)

7. Relaxation of the pelvic joints and symphysis pubis during the later months of pregnancy
   A. is caused by the increased pressure of the growing uterus
   B. is due to the hormone relaxin
   C. is due to a temporary softening of the pelvic girdle
   D. none of the above   (2:72)

8. Striae that appear on the breasts and abdomen are the result of
   A. stretching, rupture, and atrophy of deep connective tissue of the skin
   B. hemorrhagic areas
   C. high-calorie diet
   D. none of these   (6:130)

9. Which of the following is *not* a normal skin change during pregnancy?
   A. linea alba
   B. chloasma
   C. linea nigra
   D. none of the above are abnormal skin changes during pregnancy   (8:121)

10. Which of the following statements best describes the weight change that occurs in the uterus from the start of pregnancy to a term gestation?
    A. 5-fold increase
    B. 10-fold increase
    C. 15-fold increase
    D. 20-fold increase   (8:113)

11. The length of the uterus increases approximately how many times during a full term pregnancy?
    A. one
    B. two
    C. three
    D. five   (5:58)

12. The growth of the uterus during the first half of the pregnancy is accomplished through the action of
    A. the growing fetus pushing against the walls of the uterus
    B. the enlarging placenta
    C. hormonal stimulation
    D. all of the above   (8:114)

13. The growth of the uterus is due to
    A. formation of new muscle fibers
    B. enlargement of pre-existent muscles

C. both A and B
D. neither A nor B   (4:145)

14. Which muscle layer (or layers) is responsible for the constriction of the blood vessels within the uterus following childbirth?
    A. external layer
    B. middle layer
    C. internal layer
    D. all of the above   (4:145)

15. During the latter months of pregnancy the uterus is usually
    A. rotated to the left side of the woman's abdomen
    B. rotated to the right side of the woman's abdomen
    C. situated in the midline of the woman's abdomen
    D. located in any one of the above-mentioned areas   (4:145)

16. Which of the following statements best describes Braxton Hick's contractions?
    A. they begin during the early months of pregnancy, are painless, and help to enlarge the uterus
    B. they begin during the latter months of pregnancy, are uncomfortable, and help to efface the cervix
    C. they begin at the end of pregnancy, are uncomfortable, and help to dilate the cervix
    D. none of the above   (4:156)

17. Hegar's sign is a softening of the
    A. cervix at the sixth week of pregnancy
    B. vagina at the sixth week of pregnancy
    C. lower uterine segment at the sixth week of pregnancy
    D. upper uterine segment at the sixth week of pregnancy   (4:156)

18. Chadwick's sign is the result of
    A. softening of the cervix caused by increased vascularity
    B. increased vascularity in the vagina
    C. increased coloration of pigmented areas of the skin
    D. the secretory activity of the alveolar cells   (8:116)

19. Which of the following statements best describes the change that takes place in the cervix during pregnancy?

    A. harder, relatively shorter in length, larger in its diameter, increased glandular secretions
    B. softer, relatively shorter in length, longer in its diameter, increased glandular secretions
    C. softer, relatively shorter in length, shorter in its diameter, increased glandular secretions
    D. harder, relatively shorter in length, shorter in its diameter, decreased glandular secretions   (8:115)

20. Softening of the cervix occurs

    A. at conception
    B. at about the sixth week of gestation
    C. in preparation for labor
    D. at onset of labor   (5:56)

21. The glands in the cervix form a substance that is called

    A. smegma
    B. mucous plug
    C. show
    D. none of the above   (4:146)

22. Which of the following statements best describes the changes that take place in the pregnant woman's circulatory system?

    A. 50% increase in total blood volume resulting from fluid retention causes a drop in hemoglobin and hematocrit volume
    B. 30% increase in total blood volume places an increased load on the heart that reaches a peak at the end of the second trimester
    C. 30% increase in total blood volume places an increased load on the heart that reaches a peak during labor
    D. increased blood volume causes cardiac hypertrophy and a tendency to pulmonary edema during the last trimester   (4:148–9)

23. Cardiac output reaches its peak in the pregnant woman at the

    A. fifth month
    B. sixth and seventh month
    C. seventh and eighth month
    D. ninth month   (5:59)

24. At what week of pregnancy does cardiac output return to the nonpregnant levels?

    A. thirty-sixth
    B. thirty-eighth
    C. fortieth
    D. immediately after delivery   (5:59–60)

25. The total blood volume increase of 30 to 50% results in

    A. nutritional anemia
    B. pernicious anemia
    C. physiologic anemia
    D. hemolytic anemia   (5:59)

26. The minimum normal hemoglobin volume in pregnancy is

    A. 14.0 g
    B. 12.0 g
    C. 10.0 g
    D. 9.0 g   (4:148)

27. During pregnancy the vital capacity of the lungs

    A. increases
    B. decreases
    C. remains the same
    D. none of the above   (5:61)

28. Urinary frequency in early pregnancy is generally the result of

    A. pressure of the enlarging uterus on the bladder
    B. increased extracellular fluid volume
    C. a lax urethral sphincter caused by progesterone
    D. urinary infection   (4:150)

29. Urinary stasis during pregnancy is due to

    A. pressure of the gravid uterus on the ureters as they cross the pelvic brim
    B. softening of ureteral walls as a result of endocrine influences
    C. both A and B
    D. neither A nor B   (4:150)

30. During pregnancy there may be an increased tendency to excrete dextrose in the urine caused by

    A. the prediabetic state present in all pregnant women
    B. increased renal threshold for sugar in the pregnant woman
    C. reduced renal threshold for sugar in the pregnant woman
    D. none of the above   (4:150)

31. Lactosuria during the later months of pregnancy probably indicates

    A. gestational diabetes
    B. diabetes mellitus
    C. milk sugar
    D. none of the above   (4:150)

32. Gastric indigestion during pregnancy usually results from

    A. increased workload of the heart, resulting in delayed peristalsis
    B. increased stomach acidity and increased levels of chorionic gonadotropin
    C. increased peristalsis and flatulence
    D. decreased gastric motility and hypochlorhydria   (8:120)

33. During the latter weeks of pregnancy, approximately how much of the normal pregnant woman's weight gain can be attributed to extracellular fluid?

    A. 1 lb
    B. 3 lb
    C. 6 lb
    D. 8 lb   (8:122)

34. Approximately how much of the increased weight gain (during pregnancy) is lost at the time of delivery?

    A. 5 lb
    B. 11 lb
    C. 3 lb
    D. 8 lb   (8:123)

35. Approximately how much of the normal weight gain during pregnancy (22 to 26 lb) consists mainly of deposits of fatty tissue?

    A. 5 to 6 lb
    B. 2 to 4 lb
    C. 8 to 10 lb
    D. none of the above   (8:122)

36. During pregnancy the basal metabolic rate

    A. remains the same
    B. increases between 5 and 10%
    C. increases between 8 and 20%
    D. increases between 10 and 30%   (8:125)

37. Fetal heart tones usually can first be heard by the doctor or nurse at the

    A. twelfth week of pregnancy
    B. sixteenth week of pregnancy
    C. twentieth week of pregnancy
    D. twenty-fourth week of pregnancy
                                            (4:157)

38. The rate of the fetal heart during pregnancy ranges from

    A. 80 to 100/min
    B. 100 to 120/min
    C. 120 to 160/min
    D. 130 to 180/min   (4:157)

39. The rate of funic souffle is the same as that of

    A. the fetal heart sounds
    B. the uterine souffle
    C. the maternal pulse
    D. none of the above   (4:158)

40. Ballottement is possible

    A. during the earliest weeks of gestation
    B. during the fourth and fifth months of gestation
    C. at term in the primigravida
    D. during labor in the multigravida
                                            (8:128)

41. The growing uterus is usually first palpable above the symphysis pubis between the

    A. first and second months of pregnancy
    B. second and third month of pregnancy
    C. third and fourth month of pregnancy
    D. fourth and fifth month of pregnancy
                                            (4:144)

42. In determining the duration of pregnancy by measuring the height of the fundus, it is generally assumed that when the fundus is at the level of the umbilicus the woman is about

    A. four months pregnant
    B. five months pregnant
    C. six months pregnant
    D. seven months pregnant   (8:132)

43. The outline of the fetus can usually be identified by abdominal palpation by the end of the

    A. fourth month
    B. fifth month
    C. sixth month
    D. seventh month   (4:156)

44. The most common presentation is

    A. breech
    B. cephalic

C. face
D. shoulder   (4:244)

45. The amniotic fluid serves all of the following purposes *except*

A. helps to control fetal temperature
B. protects the fetus from injury
C. provides immune bodies for the fetus
D. important for fetal metabolism
                                             (8:83—4)

46. Which of the following improvements is believed to be the greatest single factor for decreasing maternal deaths during the last half century?

A. antepartal care
B. management during labor
C. care during the puerperium
D. analgesia during delivery   (4:15)

47. A primipara is a woman who

A. is pregnant for the first time
B. is in her second or any subsequent pregnancy
C. has given birth to one child of viable age
D. has not had children   (8:136)

48. A parturient is a woman

A. during the antepartal period
B. in labor
C. during the immediate postpartum period
D. during the period following her six-week postpartum period   (8:136)

49. Before attempting to accomplish Leopold's maneuvers, it is important to ask the mother to

A. assume a Sim's position
B. assume a knee-chest position
C. empty her bladder
D. bear down   (8:275)

50. In preparing the pregnant woman for pelvic examination, the nurse can be most helpful to the woman if she explains the procedure prior to the examination and then

A. instructs the patient to relax during the examination
B. responds only to direct requests for help from the woman during the examination
C. provides step-by-step guidance during the examination

D. instructs the woman that she will answer any questions following the examination   (4:175)

51. Which of the following laboratory tests could be omitted from the antepartal care routine without jeopardizing the health of the mother or fetus?

A. serologic test for syphilis
B. hemoglobin and hematocrit determination
C. blood typing and Rh determination
D. none of the above   (4:168—9)

52. Nagele's rule for calculating the estimated date of delivery states

A. determine the date of conception and count ahead 9½ months
B. count back 3 months from the first day of the last menstrual period and add 7 days
C. determine the date of quickening and count ahead 22 weeks for the primigravida and 24 weeks for the multigravida
D. determine the degree of change in the dilation and effacement of the cervix and estimate the date accordingly
                                             (5:70)

53. Symptoms one might expect a woman to notice during the first trimester of pregnancy are

A. amenorrhea, frequency, quickening
B. fullness of breasts, spotting, amenorrhea
C. frequency, morning sickness, quickening
D. fullness of breasts, frequency micturition, amenorrhea   (4:154)

54. Fatigue during early pregnancy results from

A. emotional reaction of the woman upon finding herself pregnant
B. changes in metabolism whereby sodium and water are retained and relaxation of smooth muscles occurs
C. persistent nausea and vomiting, which leave the woman exhausted
D. none of the above   (5:55)

55. During the early weeks of pregnancy the woman's usual reaction is one of

A. complete happiness at the thought of being pregnant
B. anxiety regarding her ability to become a good mother

C. concern over the ability to follow the doctor's orders during pregnancy
D. rejection of the pregnancy   (8:140)

56. The normal weight change in the first trimester of pregnancy is a
   A. gain of 0 to 3 lb
   B. gain of 3 to 6 lb
   C. gain of 6 to 10 lb
   D. loss of 3 to 5 lb   (8:123)

57. Which of the following emotional changes are considered to be normal in the pregnant woman?
   A. irritability
   B. sensitivity
   C. introspection
   D. all of the above   (8:140)

58. The usual cause of leg cramps during pregnancy is
   A. a calcium deficiency
   B. varicose veins
   C. pressure on nerves supplying the lower extremities (femoral veins)
   D. a phosphorus deficiency   (4:211)

59. Cramping in the leg can be relieved by
   A. having the mother stand up
   B. extending the leg, flexing the ankle, and forceably pushing the forefoot upward
   C. application of a hot water bottle
   D. all of the above   (8:171)

60. Which of the following is considered to be sound advice for a pregnant woman contemplating breast feeding?
   A. toward term, manually try to express up to 1 oz of milk daily
   B. cleanse nipples daily with soap to remove the oils and dried material
   C. apply a lanolin cream, massage the nipple and areola to toughen the skin
   D. wear an absorbent pad, preferably covered with plastic, in the brassiere to prevent soaking   (4:200)

61. In helping the woman with aspects relating to breast care, the nurse should
   A. instruct the woman to wear a well-fitted brassiere throughout pregnancy
   B. instruct the woman that a brassiere is necessary only if one has been worn in the past
   C. instruct the woman that a brassiere is

necessary only if she plans to breast feed the baby
   D. instruct the woman that the wearing of a brassiere really makes no difference from the physical standpoint   (4:200)

62. Which of the following signs constitute positive evidence of pregnancy?
   A. enlarging uterus, positive Aschheim-Zondek test, positive Hegar's sign
   B. positive Chadwick's sign, enlarging breasts, abdominal palpation of the fetus
   C. auscultation of FHT, x-ray visualization of the fetal skeleton, positive Hegar's sign
   D. fetal movements felt by the examiner, x-ray visualization of the fetal skeleton, and ausculation of FHT   (4:157)

63. The pregnant woman who smokes can expect that her newborn may be
   A. retarded
   B. a low-birth-weight baby
   C. premature
   D. a postmature infant   (8:155−6)

64. The effects of smoking on the unborn child have been attributed to
   A. vasoconstriction resulting in decreased placental blood flow
   B. a direct effect on fetal metabolism
   C. an increase in blood carbon monoxide level of mother and fetus
   D. all of the above   (8:155−6)

65. Which of the following symptoms is *not* caused by pressure (during pregnancy)?
   A. cramps in the legs
   B. varicose veins
   C. hemorrhoids
   D. all of the above are caused by pressure   (8:168)

66. Pressure symptoms in the pregnant woman can be prevented *most effectively* by
   A. the wearing of a maternity girdle
   B. keeping off her feet as much as possible
   C. elevation of the involved area
   D. none of the above   (8:168)

67. Swelling of the ankles is largely due to
   A. inadequate rest
   B. relaxation of the smooth muscles in the blood vessel walls
   C. decreased glomerular filtration rate
   D. increased sodium intake   (5:62)

68. The first symptom of the development of varicose veins is

    A. sharp throbbing pain in the legs
    B. areas of redness and swelling
    C. dull aching pains in the legs
    D. areas of edema   (4:209)

69. During the third trimester of pregnancy the woman's thoughts are focused primarily on

    A. her future role as wife and mother
    B. the return of her body to its pre-pregnant state
    C. general fears about the labor and delivery process
    D. all of the above   (7:40)

70. The dreams of the pregnant woman during the third trimester of pregnancy may center on

    A. the birth of an abnormal baby
    B. the birth of a stillborn infant
    C. killing the infant following the birth
    D. all of the above   (7:40)

71. Tub bathing during the latter months of pregnancy should be restricted because of the possibility of

    A. infection
    B. premature rupture of membranes
    C. slipping or falling
    D. early labor   (8:160)

72. Sexual intercourse during the last six weeks of pregnancy should be

    A. discontinued because of the possibility of infection
    B. discontinued because of the possibility of premature labor
    C. discontinued because of the possibility of placenta abruptio
    D. continued unless there are problems (8:163)

73. During the latter months of pregnancy the husband can be most helpful to his wife by

    A. ignoring her when she asks, "Do you still love me?"
    B. teasing her when she asks, "Do you still love me?"
    C. questioning her about her love for him when she asks, "Do you still love me?"
    D. responding with increased love and affection when she asks, "Do you still love me?"   (8:141)

74. Shortness of breath during the latter weeks of pregnancy can *best* be relieved by having the woman lie flat on her back with

    A. her arms at her sides
    B. her legs elevated about 55 degrees
    C. her legs elevated about 10 degrees
    D. her arms elevated above her head (8:171)

75. When a patient in the last month of pregnancy becomes pale, clammy, breathless, and hypotensive while lying on her back on the examining table, the most likely cause is

    A. abruptio placentae
    B. amniotic fluid embolism
    C. supine hypotensive syndrome
    D. syncope   (8:172)

76. Approximately two weeks before term, the primigravida experiences lightening. Body changes that often accompany this are

    A. leg cramps, urinary frequency, easier breathing
    B. abdominal pains, frequent micturition, constipation
    C. dull backaches, dyspnea, increased protrusion of the abdomen
    D. none of the above   (4:251)

77. Which of the following signs are considered to be probable signs of pregnancy?

    A. cessation of menstruation, quickening, fatigue, urinary frequency
    B. changes in the cervix, enlargement of the abdomen, Broxton Hicks contractions
    C. outline of fetal skeleton, fetal heart sounds, fetal movements felt by the examiners
    D. Chadwick's sign, fetal outline distinguished by abdominal palpation   (4:153–4)

78. "Quickening" means which of the following to a lay person?

    A. the dropping of baby into the birth canal about two weeks before term
    B. the "feeling of life" within the woman's body which is felt shortly after conception
    C. the "feeling of life" within the woman's body which is felt toward the end of the fifth month
    D. the knowledge that a child is growing within the uterus, which is affirmed by a positive pregnancy test (4:155)

79. During the middle trimester, the woman's attention is focused on
    A. her own physical condition
    B. the labor and delivery experience
    C. the new baby
    D. none of the above   (8:140)

80. During pregnancy the number of kilocalories should be increased an additional
    A. 100 per day
    B. 150 per day
    C. 200 per day
    D. 300 per day   (3:317)

81. During lactation approximately how many additional kilocalories are needed to produce enough milk to meet the daily milk requirements for the newborn?
    A. 100 kilocalories
    B. 250 kilocalories
    C. 300 kilocalories
    D. 500 kilocalories   (3:117)

82. Which of the following foods provides the highest protein value?
    A. one large egg
    B. one cup of cooked dry beans
    C. one shredded wheat biscuit
    D. one cup of milk   (3:328)

83. The calcium need during lactation is how much greater than the calcium need during pregnancy?
    A. 0.5 g
    B. 0.1 g
    C. 1 g
    D. none of the above   (3:328)

84. An adequate iron intake is needed during pregnancy to
    A. maintain the pregnant woman's hemoglobin level
    B. provide a reserve of iron for use after delivery by mother and infant
    C. furnish requirements of development for the fetus
    D. all of the above   (3:321)

85. When supplementary iron is given, the patient should be told that she might have
    A. diarrhea
    B. black stools
    C. constipation
    D. all of the above   (2:77)

86. Which one of the following provides the pregnant woman with the recommended daily amount of vitamin C?
    A. one medium-sized tomato
    B. one medium-sized orange
    C. one medium-sized potato
    D. one medium-sized banana   (3:328)

87. The pregnant woman needs an increased amount of protein for
    A. storage of nitrogen, which is essentially supplied to the uterus
    B. meeting the fetus' need for growth
    C. supplying the mammary tissue in preparation for lactation
    D. all of the above   (5:84)

88. Which of the following foods could be used as a substitute for a 2- to 3-oz serving of lean cooked meat, fish, or poultry (without bone)?
    A. half a cup of cottage cheese
    B. 4 tablespoons of peanut butter
    C. 3 oz of cheddar cheese
    D. all of the above   (4:194)

89. Which of the following foods provides the best source of iron?
    A. half a cup of carrots
    B. half a cup of orange juice
    C. 4 slices of whole wheat bread
    D. 1 cup of dried beans cooked   (3:329)

90. Which one of the following is the best source of vitamin C?
    A. half a cup of green beans
    B. half a cup of cooked cabbage
    C. half a cup of broccoli
    D. half a cup of spinach (cooked)   (3:342)

91. Approximately how much new protein is formed during the entire pregnancy?
    A. 800 g
    B. 950 g
    C. 1,100 g
    D. 1,300 g   (8:146)

92. Approximately what proportion of the newly formed protein is accumulated in the fetus?
    A. one third
    B. one half
    C. three quarters
    D. two thirds   (8:146)

93. Which of the following statements is true regarding a medium-sized apple? It produces
    A. 100 kilocalories
    B. 2 g of protein
    C. 135 IU of vitamin A
    D. 10 mg of vitamin C   (3:328)

94. One quart of milk supplies how much calcium?
    A. 0.7 g
    B. 0.9 g
    C. 1.2 g
    D. 1.5 g   (8:148)

95. Approximately what percentage of food iron intake is absorbed within the body?
    A. 5%
    B. 10%
    C. 15%
    D. 25%   (8:149)

96. Vitamin D is important for the pregnant woman because it
    A. promotes retention and utilization of calcium
    B. promotes retention and utilization of phosphorus
    C. is necessary in the formation of the bones and teeth of the fetus
    D. all of the above   (3:323)

97. Inadequate intake of folacin during pregnancy may result in
    A. pernicious anemia
    B. sickle cell anemia
    C. megaloblastic anemia
    D. none of the above   (8:151)

98. Which of the following is most likely to occur in a pregnancy where the woman had poor nutritional status *before* the pregnancy?
    A. increased pregnancy complications
    B. increased incidence of premature babies
    C. smaller babies
    D. all of the above   (2:76)

99. Which of the following is likely to occur in a woman who has a poor diet during pregnancy?
    A. premature births
    B. congenitally defective infants
    C. stillborn infants
    D. all of the above   (2:77)

100. Ascorbic acid is necessary for the pregnant woman because
    A. it increases absorption of iron
    B. it is essential for the health of gums and teeth
    C. it is necessary for the production of an intercellular substance needed for the support of cartilage, bone, muscle, and other tissues
    D. all of the above   (4:191)

101. How much ascorbic acid is recommended during pregnancy?
    A. 45 mg
    B. 60 mg
    C. 75 mg
    D. 90 mg   (3:328)

102. Although the definite cause of hyperemesis gravidarum has not been established, it has been theorized that it is due to
    A. poor nutritional status prior to onset of pregnancy
    B. physiologic changes occurring in pregnancy
    C. psychological factors associated with pregnancy
    D. both B and C   (2:121)

103. The immediate concern for a mother with severe hyperemesis gravidarum is
    A. replacement of fluid and electrolytes
    B. elimination of possible psychogenic factors
    C. consultation with a psychiatrist, since the condition most often has psychological implications
    D. impossible to determine until complete medical evaluation is made   (4:483)

104. Which of the following symptoms would indicate hyperemesis gravidarum rather than simple nausea and vomiting of pregnancy?
    A. persistent vomiting for four to eight weeks
    B. dehydration with diminished urinary output and low-grade fever, jaundice, accelerated pulse
    C. starvation with weight loss and the presence of acetone and diacetic acid in the urine
    D. all of the above   (4:483)

105. Which of the following might be used to alleviate morning nausea and vomiting without hospitalizing the patient?

A. advising her to eat a dry cracker before getting out of bed in the morning
B. psychotherapy
C. large doses of progesterone
D. none of the above (2:74)

106. The term "ectopic pregnancy" refers to the implantation of the ovum

A. in the fallopian tube
B. in the ovary
C. in the abdominal cavity
D. all of the above (4:478)

107. The symptoms of an ectopic pregnancy usually occur

A. before the first missed period
B. during the first trimester
C. during the second trimester
D. after the first missed period
(8:190−1)

108. Sometimes the first symptom of a ruptured tubal pregnancy is

A. intermittent pain in the lower abdomen with profuse vaginal bleeding
B. sudden acute pain in the lower abdomen with symptoms of shock greater than those expected with amount of vaginal bleeding
C. acute pain in the upper abdomen with symptoms of shock greater than those expected with amount of vaginal bleeding
D. profuse vaginal bleeding with expected symptoms of shock (8:190−1)

109. The most common cause of spontaneous abortion is

A. abnormalities of the ovum or sperm
B. German measles
C. abnormalities of the reproductive tract
D. systemic maternal disease (5:245)

110. Almost invariably, what is the *first* symptom of threatened abortion?

A. slight bleeding
B. severe cramping
C. mucoid discharge
D. uterine apoplexy (8:185)

111. When the fetus dies in the uterus and instead of being expelled is retained indefinitely, the situation is known medically as

A. complete abortion
B. incomplete abortion
C. missed abortion
D. none of the above (5:245)

112. If fetal weight is not known, abortion is defined as termination of pregnancy prior to

A. 12 weeks
B. 16 weeks
C. 20 weeks
D. 28 weeks (4:474)

113. A patient in early pregnancy who experiences copious bleeding and severe uterine contractions would be diagnosed as having

A. threatened abortion
B. imminent abortion
C. inevitable abortion
D. complete abortion (8:185)

114. The incidence of spontaneous abortion in all pregnancies is

A. 5 to 10%
B. 10 to 20%
C. 20 to 30%
D. 30 to 40% (8:184)

115. The term "habitual abortion" means

A. two or more consecutive spontaneous abortions
B. three or more consecutive spontaneous abortions
C. two or more spontaneous abortions
D. three or more spontaneous abortions
(2:112)

116. The most commonly accepted cause for habitual abortions during the second trimester of pregnancy is

A. nutritional deficiencies
B. incompetent cervical os
C. endocrine abnormalities
D. none of the above (4:477)

117. Preventive treatment for habitual abortions consists of reinforcing the cervix with a purse-string suture

A. at the time of the first missed period
B. at the tenth to twelfth week of gestation
C. at the fourteenth to eighteenth week of gestation
D. at the onset of dilation of the cervix
(8:189)

118. Which of the following statements is *not* consistent with the findings associated with a hydatidiform mole?

A. presence of brownish-colored bleeding starting after the twelfth week of pregnancy

B.   height of fundus larger than that expected for week of gestation
C.   well-defined fetal parts felt by abdominal palpation
D.   signs and symptoms of toxemia during second trimester of pregnancy   (5:247)

119.   A hydatidiform mole is considered
A.   a relatively common occurrence in the older pregnant woman
B.   a condition that requires both immediate and follow-up care
C.   a premalignant lesion of the decidua
D.   none of the above   (5:246–7)

120.   Although the exact cause of hydramnios is not known, this condition is most frequently seen with which of the following situations?
A.   fetal malformations
B.   excessive weight gain
C.   toxemia
D.   none of the above   (8:216)

121.   Hydramnios would be diagnosed if the amount of amniotic fluid was in excess of
A.   500 mL
B.   700 mL
C.   1,000 mL
D.   2,000 mL   (8:216)

122.   Which of the following is not considered to be a possible cause of urinary tract infections during pregnancy?
A.   drop in the number of white blood cells during pregnancy
B.   mechanical pressure on the ureters
C.   hormonal effects acting on the tonus and peristalsis of the ureters
D.   improper intestinal elimination   (4:489)

123.   Placenta previa occurs more frequently in
A.   women with toxemia
B.   multiparas
C.   primigravidas
D.   women with diabetes   (4:480)

124.   The most common cause of bleeding in early pregnancy is
A.   ectopic pregnancy
B.   placenta previa
C.   abortion
D.   hydatidiform mole   (4:480)

125.   Low implantation of the placenta is
A.   the most dangerous form of placenta previa

B.   one in which the placental margin overlaps the os
C.   not seen as a form of placenta previa
D.   none of the above   (8:193)

126.   The mother who has placenta previa will probably have a cesarean section if
A.   she is a primigravida
B.   she has a total previa
C.   there has been excessive bleeding
D.   all of the above   (4:481)

127.   Placenta previa occurs about once in every
A.   100 cases
B.   200 cases
C.   300 cases
D.   400 cases   (4:480)

128.   The *least* serious cause of bleeding in pregnancy is
A.   placenta previa and abruptio
B.   abortions and ectopic pregnancy
C.   erosions and polyps of the cervix
D.   vasa previa and hydatidiform mole   (8:193)

129.   Painless bleeding in the last trimester of pregnancy is usually caused by
A.   hydatidiform mole
B.   ectopic pregnancy
C.   placenta previa
D.   placenta abruptio   (8:193)

130.   Placenta abruptio is often associated with
A.   untreated infections
B.   Rh incompatibility
C.   cardiac disease
D.   toxemia of pregnancy   (8:196)

131.   Placenta abruptio occurs when the
A.   normally implanted placenta separates at term following the birth of the baby
B.   abnormally implanted placenta separates at term following the birth of the baby
C.   normally implanted placenta separates prematurely
D.   abnormally implanted placenta separates prematurely   (8:196)

132.   Which of the following would lead a nurse to consider that a woman had an abruptio placentae with concealed bleeding?
A.   large amount of vaginal bleeding, soft abdomen, no pain, vital signs consistent with amount of bleeding
B.   large amount of vaginal bleeding,

uterine contractions with regulation of uterus between contractions

C. small amount of vaginal bleeding, board-like abdomen, vital signs not consistent with amount of blood loss

D. small amount of bleeding, frequent uterine contractions, vital signs consistent with blood loss   (4:482)

133. What complication may occur postpartum as a result of a concealed hemorrhage in placenta abruptio?

A. hemorrhage
B. infection
C. depression
D. all of the above   (8:198–9)

134. A medication frequently given for *mild* preeclampsia is

A. magnesium sulfate
B. phenobarbital
C. soda bicarbonate
D. syntocinon   (4:467)

135. The incidence of toxemia in pregnancy is

A. less than 5%
B. between 5 and 10%
C. between 10 and 15%
D. between 15 and 20%   (4:464)

136. A diagnosis of mild preeclampsia may be made, despite a blood pressure reading of 120/80, if on two or more occasions

A. there is excessive weight gain
B. there is ankle edema
C. the diastolic pressure has risen more than 15 mm Hg and the systolic pressure has risen more than 30 mm Hg
D. there is a multiple gestation   (4:449)

137. Which one of the following is the characteristic sign that a preeclamptic woman has moved into eclampsia?

A. increasing weight gain
B. convulsions
C. decreased amount of urine
D. edema of eyelids   (8:208)

138. Which of the following drugs is most commonly used in the treatment of a woman with eclampsia?

A. magnesium sulfate
B. amytal sodium
C. morphine
D. paraldehyde   (4:471)

139. Which of the following is (are) considered to be contributing factor(s) in the etiology of toxemia?

A. stress
B. a diet high in carbohydrates and low in protein
C. impairment of uteroplacental circulation
D. all of the above   (6:175)

140. Which of the following factors are known to predispose women to the development of toxemia?

1. acute hydramnios
2. low socioeconomic level
3. diabetes with renal involvement
4. nonwhite race
5. multiple gestations

A. 1, 5
B. 1, 3, 5
C. 2, 4
D. all of the above   (6:177)

141. Death in a woman who experiences eclampsia can be due to

A. renal failure
B. cerebral hemorrhage
C. circulatory collapse
D. all of the above   (6:185)

142. What percentage of women who develop preeclampsia continue to experience hypertension following delivery?

A. 5%
B. 10%
C. 15%
D. 33%   (6:185)

143. Which of the following conditions would lead a physician to suspect that a state of prediabetes was present in a woman?

A. a past history of low-birth-weight infants
B. a past history of abortions caused by incompetent cervix
C. a past history of hypertension
D. none of the above   (6:186)

144. *Trichomonas vaginalis* is usually treated with which of the following drugs?

A. metronidazole
B. Mycostatin
C. penicillin
D. gentian violet   (8:176)

145. The *Treponema pallidum* organism should be detected during the first trimester of pregnancy because
    A. viral infections are extremely hazardous in the first trimester
    B. developmental anomalies can occur with bacterial invasion
    C. treatment instituted during the first trimester protects the infant
    D. medical history is an important factor in the over-all management of the patient (8:232)

146. Which one of the following causes of leukorrhea in a pregnant woman might cause blindness in the baby after birth?
    A. *Trichomonas vaginalis* vaginitis
    B. *Candida albicans* vaginitis
    C. gonorrheal vaginitis
    D. nonspecific vaginitis (8:233)

147. Vaginal discharge can be considered a major problem in pregnancy if
    A. it is profuse, yellow, and accompanied by burning and frequency of urination
    B. it is profuse, frothy, white or yellow, and accompanied by irritation
    C. it is profuse, cottage-cheese-like and accompanied by irritation of the vulva
    D. all of the above (4:211)

148. The malformations that most commonly result from maternal rubella during the first trimester are
    A. cataracts
    B. deafness
    C. mental retardation
    D. all of the above (8:221)

149. Sickle cell disease during pregnancy is most likely to be found in persons of
    A. Italian or Greek descent
    B. Oriental descent
    C. Negroid descent
    D. American Indian descent (2:515)

150. The sickle cell trait occurs in what percentage of American Negroes?
    A. 5%
    B. 10%
    C. 2%
    D. 15% (2:515)

151. Which of the following combinations of factors would indicate the greatest likelihood for the development of erythroblastosis fetalis?
    A. nullipara, Rh positive with Rh negative husband
    B. nullipara, Rh negative with Rh positive husband
    C. multipara, Rh negative with Rh negative husband
    D. multipara, Rh negative with Rh positive husband (8:724—7)

152. Select intrauterine transfusions are currently done
    A. whenever Rh antibodies are detected in the mother's blood
    B. when amniocentesis and a history of previous pregnancies indicate that the baby's chance for survival without treatment is extremely poor
    C. whenever there is a past history of erythroblastosis
    D. in the outpatient departments of most hospitals (4:547)

153. Which of the following statements best describes Rh negative blood?
    A. red blood cells assume abnormal shapes when oxygen tension is changed
    B. red blood cells lack a substance that is present in about 85% of people in the United States
    C. red blood cells lack a substance that is found in about 15% of the people in the United States
    D. none of the above (8:725)

154. A rising antibody titer (shown by indirect Coombs' test) on a pregnant woman indicates
    A. an infection
    B. destruction of her red blood cells by antibodies from the fetus
    C. formation of antibodies that may destroy the red blood cells of her baby
    D. an allergy to something she is eating (4:546)

155. Intrauterine death of the fetus in the mother who has been sensitized to the Rh positive factor usually results from
    A. severe anemia and circulatory collapse
    B. bilirubin pigment deposited throughout the baby, especially in the brain
    C. extramedullary hematopoiesis
    D. excessive blood volume with associated anemia (2:297)

156. A serious complication of pregnancy in which the newborn is frequently excessively large and which carries a 15 to 20% infant mortality rate is
   A. polyhydramnios
   B. hyperglycemia
   C. diabetes mellitus
   D. hypoglycemia (8:277)

157. Pregnancy is usually terminated at about the thirty-seventh week of gestation in the severe cases of diabetes because
   A. intrauterine fetal death often occurs during the last three weeks of gestation
   B. there is an increased incidence of mechanical difficulties in labor and delivery with a large baby
   C. there is an increased incidence of birth injury to the child
   D. all of the above (2:124)

158. The incidence of diabetes in all pregnancies ranges from
   A. 0.25 to 1%
   B. 0.15 to 0.75%
   C. 0.50 to 2%
   D. 1 to 2% (5:290)

159. Which of the following would be most likely to precipitate acidosis in a pregnant diabetic woman?
   A. limiting her salt
   B. decreasing her activity
   C. vomiting
   D. none of the above (5:290)

160. The discovery of sugar in the urine of a diabetic woman during pregnancy should be followed by
   A. increased insulin
   B. decreased insulin
   C. fasting blood sugars
   D. oral glucose tolerance tests (5:291)

161. Which of the following is *not* associated with diabetes in pregnancy?
   A. increased tendency to develop toxemia
   B. increased incidence of ectopic pregnancy
   C. increased incidence of hydramnios
   D. increased tendency to develop acidosis (4:488)

162. During late pregnancy the action of which of the following hormones influences the mother's need for insulin?
   1. LTH
   2. HCSM
   3. estrogen
   4. progesterone
   5. HPL
   A. 1, 2, 5
   B. 2, 3, 4
   C. 2, 3, 5
   D. all of the above (6:187)

163. Which of the following vaccinations can be safely given to a woman during pregnancy?
   1. smallpox
   2. rubella
   3. tetanus toxoids
   4. diphtheria toxoids
   5. mumps
   A. 1, 2
   B. 3, 4
   C. none of the above
   D. all of the above (3:359)

164. Who first developed a procedure by which the incompetent cervix could be reinforced by cerclage during pregnancy?
   A. Mersilene
   B. Shirodkar
   C. Lash and Lash
   D. Palmer and Lacomme (6:192)

165. Hydatidiform mole forms during what time period of the pregnancy?
   A. during the first five weeks
   B. at about the tenth week
   C. at about the twelfth week
   D. none of the above (6:193)

166. Which of the following statements *best* describes the signs and symptoms associated with hydatidiform mole?
   A. vaginal bleeding and toxemia during the first trimester
   B. hydramnios and toxemia during the second trimester
   C. vaginal bleeding and abdominal pain after the first or second missed period
   D. toxemia and enlarged abdomen during the second trimester (6:193)

167. Which of the following signs would a physician probably find while examining a woman who has a hydatidiform mole?
   A. fetal heart sounds in lower abdomen
   B. fundal size consistent with stated weeks of gestation
   C. ballottable fetus
   D. none of the above (6:193)

168. The woman who practices pica during pregnancy
    A. will probably be obese
    B. will probably have an oversized baby
    C. will probably have a premature baby
    D. will probably have a low hemoglobin level (6:160)

169. Which of the following examinations can be used to determine placental insufficiency?
    A. creatine level in amniotic fluid
    B. estriol excretion studies
    C. bilirubin level in amniotic fluid
    D. none of the above (8:234−5)

170. Which of the following groups of women can be classified under the category of high risk regarding their possible pregnancy outcomes?
    1. women in their first pregnancy
    2. women in their second pregnancy with one living child
    3. women who weigh less than 100 lb
    4. women from the low socioeconomic group
    5. women with poor reproductive histories
    A. 1, 4, 5
    B. 2, 3, 4, 5
    C. 1, 3, 4, 5
    D. all of the above (6:172)

171. Which of the following facts is most significant regarding high-risk pregnancies that result from a chronic disease?
    A. any chronic disease will put an additional burden on the woman during pregnancy
    B. any chronic disease that the woman has will be transmitted to the fetus
    C. any chronic disease that the woman has should be considered a threat to the fetus
    D. any chronic disease that the woman has may go into a state of remission during pregnancy (8:220)

Directions: Each group of numbered words or phrases is followed by a list of lettered statements. MATCH the lettered statement with the numbered word or phrase most closely associated with it.

Questions 172 through 175
172. enlargement and softening of the fundus at the site of implantation
173. a dark bluish or purplish discoloration of the mucous membrane of the lowered portion of the vagina in pregnancy
174. softening and compressibility of the lower segment of the uterus in early pregnancy
175. painless uterine contractions
    A. Braxton Hick's contractions
    B. Von Fernwald's sign
    C. Chadwick's sign
    D. Hegar's sign (6:127)

Questions 176 through 179
176. small nodular follicles or glands on the areolae around the nipple
177. a dark line appearing on the abdomen that extends from the pubis toward the umbilicus
178. the stretching, rupture, and atrophy of the deep connective tissues of the skin
179. occurrence of light brown patches of irregular shape and size on the skin of the face
    A. linea nigra
    B. Montgomery's tubercles
    C. chloasma
    D. striae gravidarum (4:147−9; 685−6)

Questions 180 through 183
180. thiazides
181. smoking
182. reserpine
183. salicylates
    A. neonatal bleeding
    B. stuffy nose with possible obstruction
    C. intrauterine growth retardation
    D. electrolyte imbalance, thrombocytopenia (8:155)

Questions 184 through 187
184. coxsackievirus
185. LSD
186. radiation
187. thalidomide
    A. midline defects of central nervous system
    B. cardiovascular anomalies
    C. phocomelia
    D. malformed legs (3:814−6)

Questions 188 through 191
188. vitamin necessary for the formation of proteins, prothrombin, and fibrin
189. vitamin that aids in the digestion of carbohydrates and an active constituent of the enzyme system
190. vitamin necessary for the growth and development of epithelial tissues and for tooth development
191. vitamin that promotes growth and proper mineralization of bones and teeth
    A. B complex group

B. D group
C. K group
D. provitamins A (6:158)

Directions: This part of the test consists of a situation followed by a series of incomplete statements. Study the situation and select the best answer to complete each statement that follows.

Questions 192 through 197
Mrs. Eleanor Jones, age 21, comes to the doctor for her first prenatal check. She states that her last regular menstrual period began on March 1 (three months ago).

192. Mrs. Jones' expected date of confinement would probably be
A. November 1
B. November 8
C. December 1
D. December 8
E. January 8 (4:115)

193. The chance that Mrs. Jones will have her baby on the calculated day is
A. less than 5%
B. less than 8%
C. less than 7%
D. less than 10%
E. none of the above (4:115)

194. Mrs. Jones states that she has also experienced nausea and vomiting and frequency of urination. These symptoms are
A. inconclusive at this time
B. indicate that a disease process has started
C. presumptive signs of pregnancy
D. probable signs of pregnancy
E. positive signs of pregnancy (5:57)

195. The doctor determines that there is a growing fetus within the uterus and states that the fundus is
A. at about the level of the symphysis pubis
B. several finger breadths above the symphysis pubis
C. on the level of the umbilicus
D. midway between the symphysis and the umbilicus
E. none of the above (4:145)

196. Which of the following statements would best describe the fetus at this time?
A. weight, 1 g; length, 30 cm
B. weight, 14 g; length, 7 cm
C. weight, 100 g; length, 15 cm
D. weight, 300 g; length, 25 cm
E. none of the above (8:102)

197. After completing the examination and finding Mrs. Jones to be a "normal patient," the doctor suggests that she return in
A. one week
B. two weeks
C. three weeks
D. four weeks
E. six weeks (8:137)

Questions 198 through 203
Ms. Jane Phillips, a 17-year-old primigravida, has been seeing the doctor regularly since her twelfth week of pregnancy. Everything appeared to be normal. Two weeks ago the following information was recorded:
32 weeks pregnant; blood pressure, 128/82; weight, 136; urine sugar negative; albumin negative; edema trace.
During today's visit, the following information was recorded on Ms. Phillips' chart:
34 weeks pregnant; blood pressure, 140/92; weight, 139; urine sugar trace; albumin trace; edema plus one.

198. Ms. Phillips is showing the signs of
A. preeclampsia, mild
B. preeclampsia, severe
C. chronic hypertension
D. diabetes mellitus
E. gestational diabetes (4:465−6)

199. Which of the following measures would the doctor probably initiate at this time?
A. sedative drugs
B. rest
C. restriction of salt in the diet
D. all of the above
E. none of the above (4:467)

200. An appropriate sedative drug for Ms. Phillips would be
A. amytal sodium
B. phenobarbital
C. magnesium sulfate
D. morphine
E. all of the above (4:467)

201. Ms. Phillips' present condition is most commonly seen in
A. young primigravidas
B. diabetics
C. chronic hypertensives

D. twin pregnancy
E. all of the above (8:202)

202. Ms. Phillips is advised to return home and

   A. take her temperature daily for fever
   B. check her weight daily for increase
   C. test her urine daily for sugar
   D. A and C
   E. B and C (4:466)

203. Ms. Phillips should

   A. return to the doctor in several days
   B. return to doctor for regular check in one week
   C. wait for two weeks before seeing the doctor again
   D. wait for the doctor to call her
   E. none of the above (4:467)

Question 204
Mr. and Mrs. Q. had planned for a baby after three years of marriage. Mrs. Q. had been to her obstetrician, who confirmed she was approximately 10 weeks pregnant. A week later she began to notice some spotting after voidings. She called her doctor, who suggested she stay on bed rest for the next 48 hours. That evening, when Mr. Q. returned from work, Mrs. Q. began to experience regular patterned contractions every 3 to 5 minutes, and the vaginal bleeding had increased. She called her obstetrician and he admitted her to the hospital.

204. Mrs. Q. was admitted because of

   A. threatened abortion
   B. inevitable abortion
   C. ectopic pregnancy
   D. missed abortion (4:474−5)

Question 205
Mrs. P., a 17-year-old primigravida, is seen in Dr. D.'s office. She states, "I just don't feel good, nurse. I feel dizzy and have been having terrible headaches this past week." On further examination the physician makes the diagnosis of preeclampsia.

205. Conditions of the patient that would indicate preeclampsia might be

   1. generalized edema
   2. increased blood pressure
   3. decreased blood pressure
   4. oliguria
   5. proteinurea
   6. convulsions

   A. 1, 2, 5
   B. 3, 4
   C. 1, 2, 4, 5
   D. all of the above (4:465−6)

Question 206
Mrs. V., a gravida I para 0, 20 years old, gives a history of having had rheumatic fever as a child with some mitral valve involvement. She visits her obstetrician after having missed two menstrual periods and he refers her for medical consultation. The consultation visit reveals a Class II functional lesion. Mrs. V. is given a 1,200-calorie low-salt diet, limitation on strenuous physical activities, and added bed rest. Her pregnancy is uneventful until at 28 weeks' gestation she experiences dyspnea and a nonproductive cough. She calls her doctor, who advises admission to the hospital.

206. The above symptoms are indicative of

   A. premature labor and delivery
   B. beginning signs of toxemia
   C. impending heart failure
   D. a beginning upper respiratory infection (4:486)

Questions 207 through 211
Mrs. Molly Jones, gravida II, para I, is a 28-year-old woman. Her obstetrical history reveals that her last pregnancy ended in spontaneous labor at the thirty-sixth week of pregnancy, followed by cesarean section after four hours of labor, because of previous surgery on her uterus. The child, a living male infant, weighed 6 lb at birth. Mrs. Jones is now in her thirty-fourth week of gestation.

207. Mrs. Jones will probably have what type of delivery with this pregnancy?

   A. normal spontaneous labor and delivery
   B. pitocin induction at thirty-eighth week of gestation
   C. trial of labor followed by cesarean section if necessary
   D. elective cesarean section (8:458)

Mrs. Jones indicated that she is afraid that she will again go into labor before the cesarean section is performed and asks how she will be able to tell that the onset of labor is approaching. Which of the following suggestions would be most helpful to Mrs. Jones?

208. Regarding vaginal secretions,

   A. there is a decrease in the amount of vaginal secretions prior to the onset of labor
   B. there is a sudden escape of a large amount of greenish secretion prior to the onset of labor
   C. there is an increase of vaginal secretions, and a small amount of blood or

"show" may be present prior to the onset of labor

    D. there is a decrease of vaginal secretions and perhaps a small amount of blood or "show" prior to the onset of labor (6:221–2)

209. Regarding weight pattern,

    A. there may be a weight gain consistent with the past pattern of gain prior to the onset of labor

    B. there may be a weight gain of 2 to 3 lb prior to the onset of labor

    C. there may be a weight loss of 2 to 3 lb prior to the onset of labor

    D. the weight may be the same as the previous week prior to the onset of labor (6:221–2)

210. Regarding the rupture of the membranes, the

    A. amniotic sac may rupture prior to the onset of labor

    B. bag of waters do not rupture prior to the onset of labor unless there is a problem

    C. membranes or bag of waters must rupture before true labor starts

    D. membranes may rupture before true labor starts (6:221–2)

211. Regarding backache,

    A. a backache at this time does not mean anything

    B. a backache at this time may indicate that the baby is lying in the wrong position

    C. a backache that persists at this time may indicate that the onset of labor is approaching

    D. a backache at this time may indicate more rest is needed (6:221–2)

Questions 212 through 215

Ms. Jenny Jones is a 19-year-old primipara and about 37 weeks pregnant. She registered at the clinic at twelve weeks of pregnancy and has been attending on a regular basis. You are assigned to be with Ms. Jones today.

212. Ms. Jones mentions that her baby is not as active as it has been in the past. Your best response would probably be

    A. we will make sure that the doctor checks the baby's heart beat today just to make sure that everything is all right

    B. when did you first notice that the baby became less active?

    C. your baby is growing very fast now and doesn't have as much room to move about in anymore

    D. usually the baby becomes less active prior to the onset of labor (6:221)

213. Ms. Jones comments that she hopes everything will be all right for her during labor. Her fears are based primarily on

    A. the movies she has seen in the past

    B. what others have told her about the labor experience

    C. her own fear of the unknown

    D. the stories her mother has told her about the experience (6:221)

214. In helping Ms. Jones you should *primarily* remember that

    A. all expectant mothers need to know a great deal of factual information about this experience

    B. each expectant mother may have different needs in regard to this experience

    C. there is certain basic information that should be given to each mother

    D. this type of information should be given to expectant mothers by the doctor (6:221)

215. Probably the best way to help Ms. Jones would be to

    A. answer only the questions that she asks

    B. assume that she is too young to know much about anything, and simply provide her with the basic information

    C. listen to what she says and provide help based on these comments

    D. find her mother and ask her how much information her daughter has received regarding labor and delivery, and go on from there (6:221)

Answers and Explanations: Antepartal Period

1. **D.** The corpus luteum maintains protection of estrogen and progesterone. In turn, the chorionic gonadotropin, secreted by the placenta, maintains the corpus luteum. High levels of estrogen and progesterone help maintain the endometrium of the uterus.

2. **D.** During pregnancy these hormones are produced by the placenta and represent the most important endocrine change during pregnancy.

3. **D.** Breast changes depend on an interaction of the hormones; the exact action is unknown.

4. **C.** Chorionic gonadotropin is produced by the trophoblastic cells of the placenta. It appears about one week after the formation of the zygote and is secreted until separation of the placenta.

5. **C.** Chorionic gonadotropin is first detected in the urine about the fifteenth day after fertilization.

6. **D.** By the third month of pregnancy the placenta assumes the production of substantial amounts of hormones and thus the role of the corpus luteum as it regresses.

7. **B.** Relaxin is an ovarian hormone.

8. **D.** The striae are believed to be the result of hyperactivity of the adrenal glands during pregnancy.

9. **D.** Skin changes during pregnancy are primarily the result of increased coloration of pigmented areas.

10. **D.** The uterus weighs approximately 2 oz (60 g) before pregnancy and approximately 2 lb (1,000 g) at the end of pregnancy.

11. **D.** The length of the uterus prior to pregnancy is 2.6 in. (6.5 cm) and approximately 12.8 in. (32 cm) at the end of pregnancy.

12. **C.** Estrogen is primarily responsible for the growth of the uterus during the first half of pregnancy.

13. **C.** The new muscle fibers strengthen the uterus for its work in pregnancy and labor. The preexisting muscles become 7 to 11 times longer and 2 to 7 times wider.

14. **B.** The muscles in the middle layer of the uterus form figure 8 fibers around the blood vessels.

15. **B.** This rotation is probably caused by the presence of the rectosigmoid on the left side of the abdomen.

16. **A.** These contractions were named after a famous London obstetrician who first described them. They are a probable sign of pregnancy.

17. **C.** Hegar's sign is a probable sign of pregnancy.

18. **B.** The normal pinkish tint of the mucous lining becomes red or purle owing to the enlarging of the blood vessels.

19. **B.** These changes are the result of an increased thickening of the mucous lining, increased blood supply, and a proliferation of the glands near the external os.

20. **B.** Softening of the cervix occurs because of congestive hyperemia of the pelvis.

21. **B.** The mucous plug forms a protective barrier against bacterial invasion of the uterus and is expelled at the onset of labor.

22. **B.** The increase in workload is no major problem for the normal heart; however, it can be a serious matter for mothers with heart disease.

23. **C.** Oxygen consumption begins at the end of the second month.

24. **C.** This fall in cardiac output prior to delivery is the result of the gradual closing down of the placental circulation.

25. **C.** The hemoglobin particles are more widely dispersed in the circulating blood.

26. **B.** Minimal hematalogic values apply to both nonpregnant and pregnant women.

27. **C.** There is a crowding of the lungs caused by fetal growth. However, the lungs increase in width and more air is inspired.

28. **A.** It appears that the growing uterus stretches the base of the bladder, creating a sensation similar to that of a stretched bladder wall.

29. **C.** Urinary stasis results when the flow of urine is impeded because of the dilated ureters and the loss of muscle tone in the ureters.

30. **C.** There is a reduction in the renal threshold for sugar frequently associated with pregnancy. Presence of sugar in the urine should be reported to the doctor.

31. **C.** Lactosuria is of no significance during the latter months of pregnancy and is due to the presence of milk sugar, which is supposed to be absorbed from the mammary glands.

32. **D.** The gastric indigestion causes heartburn and flatulence.

33. **B.** This is edema fluid.

34. **B.** During the succeeding weeks, the woman will continue to lose weight until her body returns to a close approximation of the pregnant state.

35. **A.** Excessive accumulation of fat may lead to obesity in later life.

36. **D.** The growing fetal tissue and increases in maternal tissues increase to a degree oxygen demand.

37. **C.** The fetal heart sounds may be heard by the eighteenth week of pregnancy if the abdominal wall is thin. The hearing of the fetal heart sounds constitutes a positive sign of pregnancy.

38. **C.** The usual heart rate is 140 during pregnancy.

39. **A.** Funic souffle is the soft, blowing murmur produced as the blood rushes through the umbilical cord.

40. **B.** During the fourth and fifth months of gestation, the fetus moves easily in the amniotic fluid. At this time the fetus will rebound in response to a sharp or sudden push of its examiner's finger.

41. **C.** The uterus becomes palpable above the symphysis pubis between the third and fourth month of pregnancy.

42. **C.** This method of estimating the date of confinement uses months rather than days as the unit of measure.

43. **C.** The ability to outline the fetus by abdominal palpation constitutes a probable sign of pregnancy. Occasionally, a tremor of the uterus may so mimic the fetal outline as to make this sign not sure proof of pregnancy.

44. **B.** Cephalic presentations are most common, occurring in about 97% of all deliveries at term.

45. **C.** The amniotic fluid seems to serve mainly in providing an optimal environment for the fetus during intrauterine life.

46. **A.** Antepartal care had its beginning in 1901, when pregnant women had antepartal visits from the Instructive Nursing Association of Boston.

47. **C.** This term is often used interchangeably with primigravida.

48. **B.** Parturient means bring forth young.

49. **C.** The empty bladder is a must for the woman's comfort and for the examiner's ease in palpating the abdomen.

50. **C.** Guidance given in an easy-to-understand way provides the woman with the help needed at the time needed and also diverts the woman's attention from the anticipated discomfort.

51. **D.** All of the blood tests mentioned should be performed on every pregnant woman.

52. **B.** Other ways of determining the estimated date of delivery include using the date quickening occurs, height of the fundus, size of baby on x-ray, or changes in the effacement and dilation of the cervix.

53. **D.** These are presumptive signs of pregnancy and are present during the first trimester of pregnancy.

54. **B.** Broadribb indicates that this fatigue is due to a basal metabolic rate of approximately −10.

55. **D.** The rejection is not of the baby but of the pregnancy. The baby does not become a reality until its movements are felt.

56. **A.** With an average weight gain of 24 lb for the total pregnancy, gain during the first trimester will be about 3 lb or less.

57. **D.** A degree of emotional instability is normal in the pregnant woman.

58. **C.** Other causes of leg cramps include fatigue, chilling, tense body posture, and insufficient calcium in the diet.

59. **D.** All of the methods mentioned are effective ways of relieving cramps in the leg.

60. **C.** Research indicates that use of soap may destroy the integrity of the nipple tissue. Therefore, the use of soap on the nipples should be discussed with the doctor. Lanolin creams prepare the nipple for nursing.

61. **A.** A well-fitted supporting brassiere not only relieves the discomforts that arise in the breasts during the antepartal period but also helps to prevent the subsequent tissue sagging that occurs after pregnancy.

62. **D.** These three signs are the only ones that give positive evidence of pregnancy.

63. **B.** The low-birth-weight child is one who weighs less than 5.5 lb and who suffers from the handicaps common to this group.

64. **D.** All of the factors mentioned are considered possible causes of the low-birth-weight baby.

65. **D.** Pressure symptoms during pregnancy are caused by pressure of the enlarging uterus on the veins returning from the lower part of the body.

66. **A.** The support of a well-fitting maternity girdle to the weak abdominal muscles provides relief and often prevents the occurence of pressure symptoms.

67. **B.** Edema can be relieved by elevating the feet or taking short walks to improve the circulation and prevent stasis.

68. **C.** The dull aching is due to distention of the deep vessels.

69. **C.** It is important that the nurse realize that even the well-prepared woman may have concerns about the coming delivery, and be ready to respond to these concerns in a realistic way.

70. **D.** Dreams relating to the birth of a less than perfect child are normal during the third trimester of pregnancy. When the mother actually delivers a less than perfect child, she may believe that these third-trimester dreams were actually a warning. It is important that the nurse assure the woman of the normality of such dreams and tell her that there is no relationship between them and the birth of an abnormal child.

71. **C.** During the latter weeks of pregnancy the woman may find it difficult to get in and out of the bathtub because of her large size. There is a danger of her falling and injuring herself. Therefore it is recommended she take showers or sponge baths.

72. **D.** Sexual intercourse can be continued throughout pregnancy without concern about infection or injury, as long as the couple can find a comfortable position. If the woman is prone to abortions, the doctor will probably suggest that intercourse be omitted during the first four months and perhaps throughout the total labor.

73. **D.** The woman needs extra love and attention in the form of expressions of love and extra help around the home. The extra love she receives during pregnancy will enable her to provide love to her newborn child after its birth.

74. **D.** This position enlarges the thoracic cavity to its maximum size.

75. **C.** When a woman lies on her back, the heavy uterus may press on the inferior vena cava and diminish the venous return to the heart.

76. **A.** Lightening is the settling of the unborn child's head into the pelvis, with the resulting pressure complaints.

77. **B.** The probable signs of pregnancy are observable mainly by the obstetrician after careful examination. Some of these signs are quite dependable, others may be simulated in nonpregnant conditions.

78. **C.** In early times the feeling of the baby's first movement was interpreted as the beginning of life in the unborn child. It is now known that life starts at the time of conception. The term "quickening" is still used in obstetrical terminology, whereas among the laity "feeling life" is the common synonym.

79. **C.** When the woman feels the movements of her unborn child she is ready to move her focus from herself to her baby.

80. **D.** According to the food and nutrition board of the National Academy of Science, there should be an increase of 300 kilocalories per day for the pregnant woman.

81. **D.** According to the food and nutrition board of the National Academy of Science, there should be an increase of 500 kilocalories per day to produce necessary breast milk for the newborn's requirements.

82. **B.** One cup of cooked dry beans equals approximately 16 g. Each of the other foods listed equals about 8 g.

83. **D.** The calcium needs for pregnant and lactating women are essentially the same.

84. **D.** Thus, a daily intake of 18 mg of iron is essential during pregnancy.

85. **D.** The woman will always have black or tarry stools while taking the iron pills. She may also have some type of gastrointestinal disturbance.

86. **B.** The recommended daily intake of vitamin C during pregnancy is 60 mg. One medium-sized orange supplies about 75 mg of vitamin C. One medium-sized tomato and one medium-sized potato supply about 25 mg each, and one medium-sized banana supplies about 12 mg of vitamin C.

87. **D.** During pregnancy the protein needs are increased from 55 to 65 g.

88. **D.** All of the foods mentioned in the stated amounts could be used as substitutes.

89. **D.** One cup of dried beans cooked provides 4.9 mg of iron; 4 slices of whole wheat bread provide 2.4 mg of iron; half a cup of carrots provides 0.05 mg of iron; and half a cup of orange juice provides 0.01 mg of iron.

90. **C.** One half cup of broccoli is equal to about 50 mg of vitamin C. One half cup of spinach or raw cabbage equals 25 mg, and half a cup of green beans is equal to 12 mg of vitamin C.

91. **B.** It has been estimated that approximately 950 g of new protein is formed during pregnancy.

92. **B.** Approximately half the protein formed during pregnancy is accumulated in the unborn child.

93. **C.** One medium-sized apple provides 87 kilocalories, no protein, 135 IU of vitamin A, and 6 mg of vitamin C.

94. **C.** One quart of milk supplies approximately 1.2 g of calcium.

95. **B.** Approximately 10% of the food iron that is ingested is absorbed.

96. **D.** All of the factors mentioned are considered to be functions of vitamin D.

97. **C.** Folacin deficiency may result during the last trimester of pregnancy unless the intake of folacin is adequate.

98. **D.** There is an increased incidence of all factors mentioned in women who have had poor nutritional status prior to pregnancy.

99. **D.** Studies indicate that women who have a poor diet during pregnancy have an increased rate of prematures, congenitally defective infants, and stillborn infants.

100. **D.** All of the functions stated are attributed to the action of vitamin C.

101. **B.** Approximately 60 mg of vitamin C is recommended during pregnancy. This is an increase of 5 mg over that recommended for the nonpregnant woman.

102. **D.** One theory is related to the tremendous physiologic changes that occur in pregnancy, and the other theory indicates that a neurotic factor in the woman produces the excessive vomiting.

103. **A.** The dehydration and starvation must be combatted first.

104. **D.** All of the above are part of the clinical picture of hyperemesis gravidarum.

105. **A.** The blood sugar tends to be low during pregnancy, and the disturbances in the metabolism of carbohydrates may be responsible for the nausea and vomiting. Thus, foods high in carbohydrates may help to prevent the nausea and vomiting.

106. **D.** An ectopic pregnancy is any gestation located outside of the uterine cavity, although the majority of ectopic pregnancies are located in the tubes.

107. **D.** It sometimes happens that the woman does not even realize that she is pregnant until the tube ruptures. Usually, however, she reports a missed period and slight vaginal bleeding.

108. **B.** Pain is due to the rupture of the tube. Shock is due to hemorrhage into the peritoneal cavity.

109. **A.** During the early months of pregnancy abortions are usually preceded by the death of the fetus. Fetal death, in addition to being the result of abnormalities of the ovum and sperm, is also caused by systemic maternal disease and abnormalities of the reproductive tract.

110. **A.** Bleeding with or without pain during this period can be regarded as a symptom of pending abortion and should be reported to the doctor.

111. **C.** This type of abortion is characterized by periodic spotting at the time of the monthly menstrual period and no further growth of the uterus on pelvic examination.

112. **C.** The fetus weighs approximately 400 g at the twentieth week of gestation. Thus, termination of pregnancy any time when the fetus weighs 400 g or less is defined as an abortion.

113. **B.** The abortion becomes inevitable when the membranes rupture with the resultant loss of the amniotic fluid, and cervical dilation is present.

114. **A.** About 75% of these abortions occur during the second and third months of pregnancy.

115. **B.** These abortions must be in consecutive order at approximately the same period of gestation to be termed habitual abortions.

116. **B.** The incompetent cervical os is a mechanical defect in the cervix whereby the cervical os dilates during the early months of gestation and expels the fetus.

117. **C.** This treatment has been fairly successful. The suture is removed if premature labor starts or at the end of gestation. The suture may be left in place, and the baby is delivered by cesarean section.

118. **C.** The fetal parts are not usually felt by abdominal palpation because there is usually no fetus.

119. **B.** Women who have hydatidiform moles are highly susceptible to choriocarcinomas and should be followed closely for a year following the pregnancy.

120. **A.** Hydramnios is also present in pregnancies complicated by diabetes and erythroblastosis.

121. **D.** The normal amount of amniotic fluid close to term is between 500 and 1,000 mL.

122. **A.** The other factors mentioned contribute to the incidence of urinary tract infections during pregnancy.

123. **B.** Placenta previa occurs more frequently in multiparas than in primigravidas. The specific etiologic factors are obscure.

124. **C.** The most common cause of bleeding during the early pregnancy is abortion; during the later months it is placenta previa.

125. **B.** Low implantation of the placenta is also known as marginal placenta previa.

126. **B.** In all instances of total placenta previa the woman will have a cesarean section because of complete obstruction of the birth canal.

127. **B.** It also occurs more commonly in multiparas than in primigravidas. The exact reason for this is unknown.

128. **C.** All of the other causes of bleeding indicate grave conditions during pregnancy.

129. **C.** However, the presence of pain does not rule out a central placenta previa.

130. **D.** The frequency of abruptio placentae is increased in hypertensive disease of pregnancy.

131. **C.** The hemorrhage that occurs with abruptio placentae is either external or concealed (internal).

132. **C.** The bleeding is internal, i.e., large amounts are being stored in the uterus, causing it to be tender and board-like. The blood loss can create a cause for concern for the patient's health.

133. **A.** The woman is prone to postpartum hemorrhage because the uterine muscle may have lost its ability to contract owing to dissociation of its fibers by intramuscular hemorrhage.

134. **B.** Phenobarbital 32 mg (0.5 g) can be given four times a day or twice this dosage in cases of moderate severity of the toximia.

135. **B.** Toxemia is a common complication of pregnancy.

136. **C.** A diagnosis of mild preeclampsia can be made when the previously normal blood pressure rises more than 15 mm Hg, and the systolic pressure rises more than 30 mm Hg.

137. **B.** Eclampsia is characterized by convulsions and coma and is one of the gravest complications of pregnancy.

138. **A.** Magnesium sulfate is a central nervous system depressant and therefore anticonvulsant. It is also useful in reducing blood pressure because of its relaxing effect on smooth muscle.

139. **D.** The actual origin of toxemia is still not known. Many theories have been advanced regarding contributing factors.

140. **D.** All of the complications mentioned are known to predispose women to toxemia.

141. **D.** The three primary causes of death from eclampsia are circulatory collapse, cerebral hemorrhage, and renal failure.

142. **D.** About 33% of women who have preeclampsia continue to suffer persistent hypertension.

143. **D.** The woman in a prediabetic state will usually have hydramnios, repeated abortions, history of stillborns, abnormal glucose tolerance tests, and babies with increasing birth weights.

144. **A.** The specific drug for *Trichomonas vaginalis* is metronidazole (Flagyl).

145. **C.** The spirochetes pass through the placental barrier sometime between the fifth month of gestation and the time of birth.

146. **C.** Gonorrheal vaginitis is caused by the gonococcus of Neisser, which also causes blindness in the newborn.

147. **A.** A profuse yellow discharge with accompanying urinary complications is highly indicative of gonorrhea.

148. **D.** Some studies place the incidence of congenital defects up to 25% or higher when the woman has German measles in the early pregnancy.

149. **C.** It occurs primarily in the Negro race, but it can occur in other races.

150. **B.** It occurs in about 10% of American Negroes, and there is a higher incidence in parts of Africa.

151. **D.** The Rh incompatible pregnancy results when the Rh negative woman conceives an Rh positive fetus. The Rh positive fetus may be conceived in a mating between an Rh positive man and an Rh negative woman. The Rh negative woman will begin to produce anti-Rh antibodies in response to the red blood cells of the Rh positive fetus that pass through the placental barrier into the woman's circulation. The Rh antibodies produced by the woman then pass back into the fetal circulation and combine with the Rh positive cells of the fetus and destroy them. Sensitization of the woman begins during the first Rh incompatible pregnancy in the later weeks of pregnancy and during the intrapartal period. In succeeding Rh incompatible pregnancies, the woman will produce Rh antibodies earlier in gestation and in increasing numbers. The fetus produces increased numbers of erythroblasts in response to the Rh antibodies that reach its circulatory system and destroy the Rh positive red blood cells. Thus, the problem usually increases in severity with each successive Rh incompatible pregnancy.

152. **B.** The survival rate for treated fetuses is only about 40 to 50%. However, without treatment the survival rate would be nil.

153. **B.** Rh negative blood lacks Rh antigens.

154. **C.** A positive indirect Coombs indicates that the fetus may be in danger.

155. **A.** As the rapid destruction of red blood cells in the fetus continues, the fetus develops anemia, which, if severe enough, results in heart failure and death.

156. **C.** The infant's abnormal weight is due to an excess of fat and glycogen in its body tissues.

157. **D.** All of the factors mentioned are important for the care of the woman with diabetes mellitus.

158. **A.** The severity of the disease is dependent upon the age of the woman, the duration of the disease, and the amount of renal and vascular damage present.

159. **C.** Vomiting during the first trimester of pregnancy greatly decreases the carbohydrate intake in the body. This results in problems associated with acidosis.

160. **C.** Any secretion of sugar into the urine should be followed by fasting blood sugars. Oral glucose tests during pregnancy are not accurate because of the decrease in gastric motility and delayed absorption of sugar from the intestinal tract.

161. **B.** There is no known association between ectopic pregnancies and diabetes mellitus.

162. **C.** It has been suggested that the high levels of estrogen produced during pregnancy act as an insulin antagonist. The hormones human chorionic somatomammotropin and human placental lactogen diminish the effectiveness of natural insulin. Thus, the action of these three hormones accounts in part for the increased amount of insulin a mother needs during the later part of the gestation.

163. **B.** Tetanus and diphtheria toxoids are considered to be safe for pregnant women. All other vaccinations mentioned *may* cause harm if given during pregnancy.

164. **B.** V.N. Shirodkar of India was the first man to develop a procedure by which the incompetent cervix could be reinforced by cerclage during pregnancy. Lash and Lash, and Palmer and Lacomme, recognized and treated the incompetent cervix at about the same time that Shirodkar did, but their operations were limited to the nonpregnant state.

165. **A.** Sometime between the third and fifth weeks of pregnancy, the trophoblasts can proliferate and form a mass called a hydatidiform mole.

166. **A.** The woman who has a hydatidiform mole experiences the symptoms of toxemia (during the first trimester of pregnancy) and has either intermittent or profuse vaginal bleeding.

167. **D.** There is no fetus when the condition of hydatidiform mole is present, thus there is no heartbeat and ballottement is not possible. The uterus, however, is larger than might be expected.

168. **D.** The woman who practices pica is the one who eats nonfood substances. Studies have indicated that there is a relationship between anemia and pica.

169. **B.** Loss of good placental function is reflected to some degree by the fetoplacental synthesis of estrogens. This measurement is done through the evaluation of the estriol levels in 24-hour urine specimens.

170. **C.** The women in these groups can be classified as high-risk women during their pregnancies.

171. **C.** A chronic disease condition in a woman usually produces a poor environment for the fetus

and results in a child who has not received maximum benefits during gestation. These high-risk mothers are likely to produce high-risk babies.

172. **B.** Von Fernwald's sign is the enlargement and softening of the fundus at the site of implantation. This is a probable sign of pregnancy.

173. **C.** Chadwick's sign is a discoloration of the mucous membrane of the vagina. This is a presumptive sign of pregnancy.

174. **D.** Hegar's sign is the softening of the lower uterine segment. This is a probable sign of pregnancy.

175. **A.** Braxton Hick's contractions are the painless uterine contractions that first occur at the sixteenth to eighteenth week of pregnancy. This is a probable sign of pregnancy.

176. **B.** Montgomery's tubercles are the small nodular follicles or glands on the areola around the nipple.

177. **A.** Linea nigra is the dark line appearing on the abdomen that extends from the area of the umbilicus to the mons veneris.

178. **D.** Striae gravidarum are the streaks produced by the stretching, rupture, and atrophy of the deep connective tissue of the skin.

179. **C.** Chloasma is the term given to the light brown patches of irregular shape and size that appear on the skin of the face.

180. **D.** The thiazides cause electrolyte imbalance and thrombocytopenia with possible neonatal bleeding.

181. **C.** Smoking causes intrauterine growth retardation.

182. **B.** Reserpine causes stuffy nose with possible respiratory obstruction.

183. **A.** The salicylates cause neonatal bleeding.

184. **B.** The coxsackievirus, if contracted during the first trimester of pregnancy, has been known to affect the cardiovascular system of the fetus.

185. **D.** Lysergic acid diethylamide users have been known to give birth to infants with malformed legs.

186. **A.** The infant who has been exposed to radiation during intrauterine life may have midline defects of the central nervous system as a result of this exposure.

187. **C.** Thalidomide has been known to cause phocomelia.

188. **C.** The K group of fat-soluble vitamins is necessary for the formation of protein, prothrombin, and fibrin, and also for normal clotting of the blood.

189. **A.** The B complex group aids in the digestion of carbohydrates and is an active constituent of the enzyme system.

190. **D.** The provitamins A are converted in the body to vitamin A and are essential for growth and maintenance of epithelial cells.

191. **B.** The D group promotes growth and proper mineralization of bones and teeth.

192. **D.** To determine the EDC, count back three calendar months from the first day of the last menstrual period and add seven days.

193. **A.** Less than 5% of all pregnant women go into labor on the estimated date of confinement.

194. **C.** Nausea and vomiting in early pregnancy is known as "morning sickness" and is a presumptive sign of pregnancy.

195. **A.** Mrs. Jones is about three months pregnant. The uterus rises out of the pelvis between the third and fourth month. So the fundus (or top of the uterus) will be closest to the level of the symphysis pubis.

196. **B.** The fetus by the end of the third month weighs about 14 g (1/2 oz) and is 7 cm (2.9 in.) long from crown to heel.

197. **D.** The "normal" woman will return to the doctor every four weeks until the seventh month of pregnancy, then every two weeks until the last month, and then every week until the onset of labor.

198. **A.** One or more of the symptoms (elevated blood pressure, albumin in the urine, or edema) is indicative of mild preeclampsia.

199. **D.** The doctor would undertake all of the mentioned points.

200. **B.** Phenobarbital, 1/2 gr four times a day, is the drug of choice in preeclampsia, mild.

201. **E.** Toxemia is seen fairly commonly in young primigravidas, in diabetics, in chronic hypertensives, and in twin pregnancies.

202. **B.** One of the most promising prophylactic measures is the curtailment of weight gain.

203. **A.** Ms. Phillips should be seen at least twice a week by the doctor.

204. **B.** Mrs. Q. is now experiencing the symptoms associated with an inevitable abortion. The process of labor has started, and a vaginal exami-

nation would probably reveal that dilatation has started.

205. **A.** The characteristic signs and symptoms of preeclampsia are: 1) generalized edema that is most evident in excessive weight gain, 2) sudden onset of high blood pressure, and 3) the appearance of albumin in the urine.

206. **C.** Mrs. V. is showing signs and symptoms of heart failure. These include, in addition to those already mentioned, a sudden limitation in the woman's ability to continue with her usual activities.

207. **D.** Mrs. Jones should have an elective cesarean section because of twice repeated surgery on the uterus. Although she delivered s small baby previously, she has never delivered a child via the vaginal route.

208. **C.** Prior to the onset of labor, vaginal secretions increase in amount, and the operculum that occluded the cervical canal may escape. This mucus mixed with a small amount of blood is termed "show."

209. **C.** Prior to the onset of labor, there may be a weight loss of 2 to 3 lb. This loss is caused by excretion of body water.

210. **D.** The membranes may rupture before true labor starts. Mrs. Jones may not know what "amniotic sac" means and become frightened, believing this to be part of the uterus.

211. **C.** A backache that persists at this time may indicate that labor is approaching.

212. **C.** During the latter weeks of pregnancy, the child is attaining full growth, and there is a lessening amount of space in the uterus.

213. **C.** All women have general concern for their labor and delivery experience. One of the primary concerns is fear of the unknown.

214. **B.** Each woman has been exposed to a unique set of past experiences and thus has different needs in regard to the present labor and delivery experience.

215. **C.** You must be able to hear what Ms. Jones is saying and respond to her concerns in order to be a truly helping person.

CHAPTER 5

Intrapartal Period

The presence of a nurse in the labor and delivery room can provide utmost support to a woman and her husband during this stressful time.

Information on the normal and abnormal aspects of the parturition period are included within this chapter. Included also are questions on fetal monitoring and its implications for the pregnancy outcome.

As in the other chapters that deal directly with childbearing and childrearing, there are situational questions at the end of the chapter.

The therapeutic role of the nurse in labor and delivery cannot be emphasized enough. Appreciation of the problems involved will allow for the satisfaction that comes from service in this area of nursing.

Directions: Each of the questions or incomplete statements below is followed by four suggested answers or completions. Select the BEST answer in each case.

1. Which of the following factors regarding the initiation of labor is most generally accepted?
   A. uterine stretch theory
   B. oxytocin theory
   C. lowering of progesterone levels
   D. all of the above   (2:130)

2. The normal range of the fetal heart is
   A. 110 to 140 beats/min
   B. 120 to 160 beats/min
   C. 120 to 180 beats/min
   D. 100 to 160 beats/min   (4:316)

3. In the passage through the birth canal, the presenting part of the fetus undergoes certain positional changes that constitute the mechanism of labor. These movements are designed chiefly to
   A. present the smallest possible diameters of the presenting part to the irregular shape of the pelvic canal, so it will encounter as little resistance as possible
   B. present the anterior-posterior diameter of the fetal skull so it will accomplish the process of cervical dilation more efficiently
   C. present the smallest possible diameters of the fetal skull to the irregular dimension of the outlet so that the occiput will present in the posterior position
   D. present the largest diameters possible so that the following diameters of the fetus will pass through the birth canal more easily   (8:299)

4. Meconium-stained amniotic fluid during labor is usually indicative of
   A. transition
   B. uteroplacental insufficiency
   C. toxemia
   D. fetal distress   (8:365)

5. The shortening of the cervical canal from a structure of 1 to 2 cm in length to one in which no canal exists but merely a circular orifice with almost paper-thin edges is known as
   A. dilatation
   B. labor

C. effacement

D. engagement   (8:292−3)

6. After the birth of the fetal head, it remains in the anterior-posterior position only a very short time and shortly will be seen to turn to one side or the other of its own accord. This maneuver (or mechanism) is known as

A. internal rotation

B. extension

C. expulsion

D. external rotation   (6:244)

7. During labor, the pregnant patient receiving insulin will have to be watched carefully for

A. hyperglycemia

B. precipitate delivery

C. hypertension

D. hypoglycemia   (8:226)

8. Which of the following drugs might be used for analgesia during labor?

A. meperidine hydrochloride

B. scopolamine

C. atropine

D. phenobarbital   (4:290)

9. By definition, a low forceps delivery is performed only when the

A. presenting part is on the pelvic floor and the cervix is fully dilated

B. presenting part is at station 0 and the cervix is effaced

C. oncoming fetal head is unable to pass through the pelvic inlet

D. oncoming head is in a persistent posterior lie   (8:450)

10. The anterior fontanel of the fetus

A. is called the "soft spot" and is formed by the parietal and frontal bones

B. is triangular and useful in determining the relative degree of rotation of the fetal head

C. is formed by the lambdoidal suture and the temporal bones

D. can become depressed in the presence of newborn intracranial bleeding   (8:259)

11. In general, when is it usually safe to administer a narcotic analgesic to a patient in labor?

A. during the first 4 cm of dilation

B. during the stage of transition

C. after 4 to 5 cm of dilation

D. during the last 4 cm of dilation   (8:314)

12. "Station" refers to the relationship of the presenting part to the mother's

A. linea terminalis

B. ischial spines

C. perineum

D. ischial tuberosity   (8:273)

13. A complete breech means that

A. one or both feet present

B. buttocks present; legs are extended and lie against the abdomen and chest

C. buttocks and feet present; legs and feet are flexed on thighs and thighs are flexed on abdomen

D. the scapula presents   (8:266)

14. Partial effacement takes place during the latter weeks of pregnancy as a result of the action of

A. progesterone

B. estrogen

C. the engaging head

D. Braxton Hicks contractions   (8:293)

15. Sparteine sulfate (Tocasamine) is used primarily

A. to aid in separation of the placenta from the uterine wall

B. to control bleeding following separation of the placenta

C. to hasten involution during the postpartum period

D. to induce labor   (4:336)

16. Which of the following drugs is generally utilized to produce long-lasting uterine contractions during the postpartum period?

A. ergotrate

B. pitocin

C. syntocinon

D. none of the above   (6:248)

17. The average amount of blood loss during a spontaneous, vaginal delivery is

A. 100 mL

B. 300 mL

C. 500 mL

D. 1,000 mL   (4:503)

18. Immediately following the rupture of the amniotic membranes, the nurse should

A. check consistency of contraction

B. wash the perineum and provide a dry pad

C. notify the physician and record the information

D. check fetal heart rate   (8:372)

19. The first stage of labor is known as the stage of
    A. dilatation
    B. expulsion
    C. placental separation
    D. recovery   (8:285)

20. The average length of the total labor in the primiparous woman is
    A. 8 to 9 hours
    B. 10 to 11 hours
    C. 12 to 13 hours
    D. 14 to 15 hours   (8:285)

21. The average length of the expulsive stage in the multigravida is
    A. 15 minutes
    B. 30 minutes
    C. 45 minutes
    D. 60 minutes   (8:285)

22. Which of the following are considered to be premonitory signs of labor as experienced by the woman?
    A. lightening
    B. false labor pains
    C. show
    D. all of the above   (8:286)

23. The settling of the fetal head into the brim of the pelvis, which may occur at any time during the last several weeks or during labor, is
    A. lightening
    B. effacement
    C. dilatation
    D. quickening   (8:286)

24. Contractions that occur irregularly, do not appear with increasing frequency, and do not increase in intensity are usually indicative of
    A. onset of true labor
    B. false labor pains
    C. behavior experienced more often in the primigravida than in the multigravida
    D. none of the above   (8:287)

25. Show is caused by
    A. separation of the placenta prior to the onset of labor
    B. separation of superficial mucosa of the cervical canal
    C. rupture of a varicosity on the external genitalia
    D. rupture of a marginal sinus   (8:287)

26. False labor contractions may begin
    A. three to four weeks before onset of labor
    B. two to three weeks before onset of labor
    C. one to two weeks before onset of labor
    D. hours before onset of labor   (4:251)

27. During the latter weeks of pregnancy, the Braxton Hicks contractions of pregnancy may reach an intrauterine pressure of
    A. 5 to 10 mm Hg
    B. 20 to 40 mm Hg
    C. 1 to 2 mm Hg
    D. 25 to 45 mm Hg   (8:292)

28. In describing the characteristics of a uterine contraction, one might say that the increment phase
    A. occurs at the middle of the contraction
    B. is about the same length as the acme phase
    C. occurs at the end of the contraction
    D. is longer than both the acme and decrement phase   (4:254)

29. Generally speaking, the primigravida should come to the hospital when her contractions
    A. first start to cause her discomfort
    B. are regular regardless of the frequency
    C. are regular and about 15 minutes apart
    D. are regular and about 5 to 8 minutes apart   (6:222)

30. The onset of labor is said to occur when the musculature of the uterus starts
    A. painful contractions and brings about the start of cervical effacement
    B. true pronounced contractions and brings about the progressive cervical effacement and dilatation of the cervix
    C. regular uterine contractions and brings about effacement of the cervix
    D. contractions that bring about some effacement and dilatation of the cervix   (6:242)

31. Rupture of the membranes prior to the onset of labor *usually* indicates that labor will
    A. begin within 24 hours
    B. be prolonged
    C. be complicated by infection
    D. be rapid   (8:288)

32. The color of amniotic fluid under normal conditions is

A. yellow
B. port-wine colored
C. clear
D. brownish   (8:288)

33. Which of the following statements describes the pattern of normal uterine contractions during early labor?

   A. occurring at 2- to 4-minute intervals, lasting 50 to 60 seconds
   B. occurring at 10- to 20-minute intervals, lasting 15 to 30 seconds
   C. occurring at 50- to 60-second intervals, lasting 1 to 2 minutes
   D. occurring at 2- to 3-minute intervals, lasting 2 minutes   (8:290−1)

34. At the peak of a normal uterine contraction, the intrauterine pressure may be from

   A. 10 to 15 mm Hg
   B. 15 to 25 mm Hg
   C. 35 to 60 mm Hg
   D. 50 to 70 mm Hg   (8:291−2)

35. Which of the following tests is used to determine the pressure of ruptured membranes?

   A. Guthrie assay test
   B. gravindex test
   C. Nitrazine test
   D. pregnosticon test   (8:289)

36. Cervical dilation is the process by which the

   A. cervical canal enlarges as the baby engages itself in the birth canal
   B. cervical canal becomes completely obliterated
   C. external os of the cervix enlarges to about 5 cm in diameter
   D. external os of the cervix enlarges enough to permit the baby's head to pass through it   (8:293)

37. At the onset of labor in the primigravida, the external os of the cervix is usually

   A. closed or slightly less than 1 cm
   B. 1 cm dilated
   C. 2 cm dilated
   D. 5 cm dilated   (8:294)

38. Effacement in the primigravida

   A. precedes dilatation
   B. occurs concurrently with dilatation
   C. occurs following dilatation
   D. is never really complete   (6:243)

39. The transition phase of labor occurs from

   A. onset of labor to 4-cm dilatation of cervix
   B. 4-cm dilatation to 7-cm dilatation of cervix
   C. 7-cm to complete dilatation of cervix
   D. full dilatation of cervix to delivery of the infant   (6:285)

40. During the latent phase of labor

   A. dilatation progresses rapidly
   B. effacement primarily occurs
   C. the head descends into the birth canal
   D. none of the above   (8:295)

41. Oozing of blood during the active phase of the dilatation stage of labor is usually due to

   A. abruptio placenta
   B. marginal placenta previa
   C. stretching and slight tearing of the cervix
   D. none of the above   (8:296)

42. The active phase of labor begins when the cervix is

   A. 2 to 3 cm dilated
   B. 3 to 4 cm dilated
   C. 6 to 7 cm dilated
   D. 7 to 9 cm dilated   (8:295)

43. The second stage of labor is known as the

   A. stage of placental separation
   B. stage of expulsion
   C. stage of recovery
   D. none of the above   (8:285)

44. The child's birth is accomplished through the assistance of

   A. uterine muscle contractions
   B. abdominal muscle contractions
   C. both A and B
   D. neither A nor B   (8:297)

45. "Crowning" occurs when

   A. the largest diameters of the baby's head have passed through the pelvic inlet
   B. the largest diameters of the baby's head have passed through the pelvic outlet
   C. the largest diameters of the baby's head are encircled by the vaginal opening
   D. none of the above   (8:299)

46. Which of the following is *not* a sign of placental separation?

   A. uterus becomes discoid in shape
   B. controlled bleeding from the vagina

C. fundus rises to the level of the umbilicus

D. umbilical cord lengthens (8:308)

47. Which of the following is *not* associated with the Schultz mechanism?

A. bleeding usually follows delivery of placenta

B. placenta becomes inverted on itself during delivery

C. rough maternal surface is presenting part of placenta

D. separation takes place first in the middle of the placenta (8:309)

48. Which of the following terms apply to the intrapartal period?

A. accouchement

B. parturition

C. confinement

D. all of the above (4:251)

49. The transitional stage lasts approximately how long in the primigravida?

A. 15 minutes

B. 30 minutes

C. 45 minutes

D. 1 hour (4:268)

50. Which of the following signs and symptoms generally indicate that the woman is in the transitional stage?

A. nausea, hiccoughs, sense of panic

B. excitement, slight anxiety

C. dull, dragging pains felt in lower back, abdomen, and thighs

D. all of the above (4:309)

51. The term "attitude" in obstetrical terminology refers to the

A. relationship between a specific, yet arbitrary point on the presenting part of the fetus to the four quadrants of the maternal pelvis

B. relation of the fetal members to each other in the uterus

C. relation of the long axis (spine) of the mother to the long axis of the fetus

D. woman's posture during pregnancy (2:129)

52. The fourth stage of labor has been defined as the time following the delivery of the placenta through the first

A. 30 minutes postpartum

B. 60 minutes postpartum

C. 10 days postpartum

D. 6 weeks postpartum (6:278)

53. The term "ripe cervix" is used to describe the cervix

A. during the early weeks of pregnancy

B. at term

C. at full dilation

D. at the end of the postpartum period (3:435)

54. When the undelivered head has descended to the perineum it is at what station?

A. +1

B. +2

C. −1

D. −2 (3:425)

55. Which one of the following methods of induction is most frequently used at term with a living baby?

A. administration of prostaglandins

B. rupture of the membranes

C. intravenous oxytocic drugs

D. stripping of the membranes (3:438−40)

56. When providing care for a woman receiving a medical induction, which of the following should be reported to the doctor?

A. contractions lasting 40 seconds

B. contractions lasting 70 seconds

C. contractions occurring every 2 minutes and lasting 90 seconds

D. none of these (4:457)

57. The basal fetal heart rate is most *accurately* the rate recorded

A. prior to the onset of labor

B. immediately prior to each contraction

C. between each contraction

D. in the intervals between the various normal periodic fetal heart rate changes (8:351)

58. The normal basal fetal heart rate is

A. between 115 and 155 beats/min

B. between 120 and 150 beats/min

C. between 125 and 155 beats/min

D. between 130 and 160 beats/min (8:353)

59. Which of the following cannot usually be determined by intermediate stethoscopic monitoring?

A. general estimate of fetal position

B. number of fetal heart beats per minute

C. quality of fetal heart beats per minute

D. normal baseline fluctuations (8:351)

60. When using a stethoscope to record fetal heart rates during labor, which of the following would *not* be consistent with a normal fetal heart rate?

    A. basal rate between 125 and 155 beats/min
    B. no significant change in basal rate throughout labor
    C. a slowing of the rate during contractions
    D. no slowing of the rate following contractions   (8:355)

61. Electronic devices in obstetrics are essential for determining

    A. frequency, intensity, and duration of contractions
    B. continuous recordings of fetal heart patterns
    C. both A and B
    D. neither A nor B   (3:442)

62. If the fetal heart rate drops during labor, which of the following actions should be taken *first?*

    A. administering oxygen to the woman
    B. turning the woman on her side
    C. calling the doctor
    D. elevating the head of the bed   (2:145)

63. Which one of the following drugs, given during labor, has an action similar to that of morphine but is less potent and less depressing and has a shorter action?

    A. Demerol
    B. Nisentil
    C. leritine
    D. scopolamine   (8:314)

64. Demerol should be avoided

    A. during the active stage
    B. when the woman wishes to remain in control of her actions
    C. late in labor
    D. when Phenergan has been administered previously in the same labor   (4:228)

65. When is the best time to give the woman pentobarbital sodium?

    A. early in labor
    B. immediately prior to delivery
    C. during the active stage
    D. it should not be given during labor   (4:290)

66. Protection from self-injury should be provided for the woman in labor who receives

    A. seconal sodium
    B. scopolamine
    C. Largon
    D. leritine   (4:291)

67. Which anesthesia is preferred when the woman is emotionally and physically able to participate completely in the birth of her child but will have an episotomy done prior to the birth?

    A. local infiltration
    B. pudendal block
    C. paracervical block
    D. caudal anesthesia   (4:291)

68. The paracervical block is an infiltration of a local anesthetic into the

    A. pudendal nerves
    B. pelvic plexus
    C. subarachnoid space
    D. epidermal space   (8:321)

69. The paracervical block provides relief of pain in the

    A. perineum and vulva
    B. uterus and cervix
    C. pelvic region
    D. T-9 to T-11   (8:321)

70. Which of the following can be given to the woman during the active phase of labor?

    A. spinal
    B. saddle block
    C. epidural
    D. pudendal block   (8:325)

71. Which of the following would indicate that the doctor has been successful in his efforts to inject local anesthetic solution in the caudal space?

    A. patient's feet become warmer and dry
    B. patient has difficulty moving legs
    C. patient has sudden, mild headache
    D. all of the above   (4:292–3)

72. When Pentrane is being utilized as a self-administered analgesic, which of the following signs would indicate that the woman is inhaling too much gas?

    A. increase in blood pressure
    B. decrease in blood pressure
    C. slow pulse rate
    D. decreased urinary output, rapid respirations   (8:317–8)

73. The anesthesia of choice for the woman whose unborn child is in the breech position would probably be

    A. caudal
    B. spinal
    C. epidermal
    D. none of the above   (4:298)

74. One of the major problems associated with spinal anesthesia is

    A. hypertension
    B. hypotension
    C. fetal bradycardia
    D. fetal tachycardia   (4:296)

75. Who first used anesthesia in obstetrical practice?

    A. Shippen
    B. Van Deventer
    C. Simpson
    D. Channing   (8:312)

76. The occiput is used in defining fetal position. It is located

    A. behind the small fontanel
    B. between the two fontanels
    C. to the sides of the large fontanel
    D. in front of the large fontanel   (8:260)

77. The most accurate way to evaluate the uterine contractions during labor is to

    A. watch the woman's reaction
    B. ask the woman about the contractions
    C. ask the husband to time the contractions
    D. time them yourself   (3:435—6)

78. The intensity of the contraction is best determined by

    A. asking the woman about the degree of discomfort she is experiencing with each contraction
    B. indenting your fingers into the uterus during the height of each contraction
    C. keeping your fingers lightly on the fundus
    D. all of the above   (4:315)

79. The nurse should check the maternal pulse at the same time she listens to the fetal heart beat primarily

    A. because rapid pulse may influence the fetal heart rate
    B. because a slow pulse is consistent with a slow fetal heart rate

    C. to make sure she is not listening to the uterine souffle
    D. none of the above   (3:436)

80. Which of the following is generally to be expected in a woman laboring with a breech presentation?

    A. she may have a longer labor than the woman with a vertex presentation
    B. she may have a more painful labor than the woman with a vertex presentation
    C. she may have a somewhat harder delivery of the after-coming head
    D. she may have more bleeding than the woman with the vertex presentation   (3:467)

81. Once the membranes have ruptured, the laboring woman, generally speaking,

    A. must stay in bed to prevent infection
    B. must stay in bed because of the possibility of a rapid dilation
    C. may be up providing there is a perineal pad between her legs to absorb the leaking fluid
    D. may be up if the presenting part fits snugly in the pelvis and is well applied against the cervix   (3:468)

82. When the vertex is in a posterior position, it may be helpful to

    A. have the woman lie flat on her back
    B. have the woman lie on her left side
    C. have the woman lie on her right side
    D. have the woman lie on the side opposite the infant's back   (3:474—5)

83. Which of the following measures can be of help in relieving cramping of the legs during the second stage of labor?

    A. having the mother wear leg stockings
    B. straightening the leg and applying pressure to the ball of the foot
    C. asking the mother to relax
    D. none of the above   (6:270—1)

84. During active labor when the woman cries, "Don't touch me, get out" or similar statements, the nurse should

    A. ask the woman why she feels this way
    B. leave the room at once
    C. stay with her
    D. find another nurse to stay with the woman   (3:447)

85. The purpose of the wrist cuffs which the woman wears during the delivery process is to
    A. protect the woman from thrashing about during the actual delivery
    B. protect the staff from the woman's aggressive actions
    C. protect the woman from injury
    D. all of the above   (6:271)

86. During the delivery room experience, the nurse can *best* support the woman by
    A. constantly talking to her while she (the nurse) moves around the room
    B. remaining silent so that the woman can rest between contractions and can concentrate all her efforts on pushing during the contractions
    C. talking slowly and exactly into the woman's ear, assuring her that she is doing well
    D. ignoring the woman while at the same time continuing conversations with other staff members in the delivery room   (3:469)

87. Lifting the woman's legs simultaneously for placement in the stirrups
    A. reduces discomfort for the woman
    B. helps to prevent an uncontrolled delivery of the infant's head
    C. makes it easier to place the legs in the stirrups
    D. prevents straining of the pelvic ligaments   (4:330−1)

88. During the entire childbearing process, which of the following is considered by the parents to be the most critical period for the parents?
    A. antepartal
    B. intrapartal
    C. immediate postpartal
    D. late postpartal   (4:299)

89. In providing effective nursing care to the woman and unborn child during the laboring process, the father should
    A. not be allowed to participate at all
    B. be allowed to visit with the woman when she requests it
    C. be allowed to visit with the woman when he requests it
    D. be allowed to participate to the degree to which he is able and can derive a sense of satisfaction from it   (4:299)

90. Usually, vital signs should be taken how often during the laboring experience?
    A. every half hour
    B. every hour
    C. every four hours
    D. every eight hours   (4:310)

91. The degree to which the nurse will use physical contact as part of her supportive care during labor will depend on the
    A. gravida of the woman
    B. phase of labor
    C. presence or absence of the husband in the labor room
    D. individual patient   (4:312)

92. The perineal shave is done for which of the following reasons?
    A. more adequate skin preparation prior to delivery
    B. easier repair of the perineal area
    C. better cleaning of the perineal area during postpartum period
    D. all of the above   (8:333)

93. The woman is instructed not to eat when she goes into labor because
    A. she may be excited or nervous, and eating at this time may give her indigestion, which will produce additional discomfort during labor
    B. full or partial energy resources will be directed toward digestive processes, and active labor will not progress
    C. digestive processes are speeded up during labor, and the woman may have excessive fecal material in the rectal region at delivery
    D. digestive processes are slowed or even stopped during labor   (8:336)

94. Which of the following would contradict the routine admission order of an enema?
    A. inactive labor
    B. ruptured membranes and engaged head
    C. vaginal bleeding
    D. early active labor   (8:333)

95. Low backache during labor may best be relieved by
    A. having the mother turn on her side during the contraction
    B. gentle massage in the lower back area
    C. firm massage or pressure on the lower back area
    D. heating pad to the lower back area   (8:347)

96. Voluntary pushing during the latter part of the active phase of labor may result in
    A. delivery of the infant
    B. full dilatation of the cervix
    C. edema of the cervix
    D. none of the above (8:348)

97. Which of the following symptoms during labor might indicate that toxemia is developing in the woman?
    A. flushed face
    B. headache
    C. cramps in legs
    D. none of the above (8:350)

98. Which of the following vaginal discharges should be reported to the doctor?
    A. mucoid material with small amounts of blood
    B. clear fluid
    C. trickle of bright red blood
    D. none of the above (8:350)

99. A third-degree laceration is one which
    A. extends only through the fourchette
    B. involves the muscles of the perineal body
    C. extends entirely through the perineal body and through the rectal sphincter
    D. results in tearing in the labia or around the urethra (8:387)

100. Immediately following the birth of the baby's head, the doctor will
    A. perform the Crede treatment
    B. check the baby's head for possible abnormalities
    C. check to see whether the cord is around the baby's neck
    D. do the Apgar rating (8:388)

101. During labor the woman may cry out for her mother. The nurse should
    A. tell the woman that she is mature enough to cope with the situation without her mother
    B. recognize that this woman is immature and remain with her to provide necessary support
    C. leave the room, recognizing that she cannot provide the kind of support the woman desires at this time
    D. recognize that the woman is indicating her need for a significant person to be on hand and remain with her to provide support (7:102)

102. Which of the following attitudes would indicate that the laboring woman is progressing into the active stage of labor (4 to 8 cm)?
    A. excitement; happiness
    B. apprehension; desires to have someone remain with her
    C. irritability; does not wish to be touched
    D. eager to be "put to sleep" (2:142)

103. A tetanic contraction is one which
    A. lasts less than 15 seconds
    B. has 2 or more peaks
    C. lasts 2 minutes or more
    D. causes no discomfort to the woman (2:146)

104. Women who are prepared in the Lamaze method of natural childbirth will probably use which of the following breathing patterns during early labor?
    A. slow, deep chest breathing
    B. long, slow, deep abdominal breaths
    C. relaxation and abdominal breathing
    D. slow, even pant breathing (8:343)

105. Which mechanism of labor is responsible for the delivery of the fetal head?
    A. extension
    B. restitution
    C. external rotation
    D. expulsion (6:244)

106. During extension, the major resistance is that of
    A. cervix
    B. pelvic floor
    C. bony pelvis
    D. uterine muscles (8:320)

107. What maneuver is performed during delivery to control the delivery of the head in the normal spontaneous delivery?
    A. Leopold's maneuver
    B. Ritgen's maneuver
    C. Mauriceau maneuver
    D. Scanzoni maneuver (6:245)

108. During the delivery of the head, the woman may be asked to
    A. pant during the contractions
    B. push during the contractions
    C. do accelerated and decelerated breathing during the contractions
    D. none of the above (8:385–6)

109. Following the delivery, the mother should first see her baby
  A. in the delivery room
  B. at the end of the fourth period of labor
  C. when she is settled down in the post-partum unit
  D. at the first feeding period following the child's birth (8:419)

110. When the newly delivered mother develops chills during the fourth period of labor, it is usually caused by
  A. infection
  B. loss of excessive amount of blood
  C. oxytocic drugs
  D. unknown factors (3:510)

111. The process by which the doctor applies pressure to the abdomen between the fundus and the symphysis with one hand and applies traction to the cord of the placenta with the other hand is known as
  A. Crede's method
  B. Schultz mechanism
  C. Brandt-Andrews' maneuver
  D. none of the above (6:246)

112. In using the nitrazine test to determine the presence of ruptured membranes, the test paper will be
  A. yellow to olive-green
  B. green to red
  C. blue-green to deep blue
  D. none of the above (6:253)

113. In the internal system of fetal monitoring
  1. a teflon catheter is placed within the uterine cavity
  2. transducers mounted in a capsule are strapped to the woman's abdomen
  3. a small electrode is clipped to the presenting part of the fetus
  4. a transmitter is introduced into the uterus
  5. a doptone is used
  A. 1, 2
  B. 1, 3
  C. 2, 4
  D. none of the above (6:257—8)

114. During labor, the nurse should avoid the word pain in connection with uterine contractions because
  A. uterine contractions are not painful
  B. uterine contractions are painful, but the nurse should not mention this to the laboring woman
  C. of the very connotation of the word
  D. the woman who is having natural childbirth cannot have medication for the pain (4:313)

115. The normal blood fibrinogen level during pregnancy is
  A. 50 to 100 mg/dL
  B. 150 to 200 mg/dL
  C. 250 to 500 mg/dL
  D. 600 to 650 mg/dL (6:129)

116. Which of the following are considered to be advantages of delivery in a recumbent position?
  A. the woman avoids the use of the rigid stirrups
  B. there is no pressure on the inferior vena cava from the uterus
  C. if vomiting occurs, there is less danger of aspiration
  D. all of the above (6:271)

117. Dystocia is a difficult labor resulting from
  A. poor nutritional status
  B. poor maternal health
  C. faults in mechanical factors involved in the birth process
  D. abruptio placentae (8:431)

118. Uterine dysfunction is caused primarily by
  A. overdistention of uterus
  B. maternal age
  C. injudicious use of analgesia
  D. premature labor (4:494)

119. Dysfunctional labor occurs when labor is prolonged during which phase?
  A. latent
  B. active
  C. fetal descent
  D. all of the above (8:431)

120. Dysfunctional labor is most likely to occur when which of the following is present?
  A. a low-birth-weight baby
  B. a premature baby
  C. a normal-sized baby
  D. an excessively large baby (4:494)

121. Which of the following is *not* associated with hypertonic uterine dysfunction (or primary inertia)?
  A. prolonged latent phase of labor
  B. contractions become infrequent and of poor quality
  C. does not respond favorably to oxytocin
  D. sedation helps a great deal (2:194—5)

122. The treatment of hypertonic uterine dysfunction is
    A. cesarean section
    B. stop labor and provide rest
    C. stimulation of labor and give fluids
    D. none of the above   (2:194—5)

123. Which of the following signs would generally indicate that complications might be occurring as a result of uterine dysfunction?
    A. excessive internal bleeding
    B. bladder distention
    C. elevation of temperature and pulse
    D. hyperactivity of the patient   (4:494)

124. A precipitous labor and delivery is one
    A. of three hours or less
    B. of two hours or less
    C. in which the baby is born unattended anywhere, but in the delivery room
    D. in which the baby is born in the delivery room without the assistance of the doctor   (8:435)

125. Premature rupture of membranes occurs more frequently in which of the following cases?
    1. ROA
    2. ROP
    3. LSA
    4. LSP
    5. multiple pregnancies

    A. 1, 3, 5
    B. 2, 4, 5
    C. 2, 3, 4, 5
    D. all of the above   (6:302)

126. A premature labor is one that occurs between
    A. the twentieth and thirty-eighth week of gestation
    B. the twenty-second and thirty-eighth week of gestation
    C. the twenty-fourth and thirty-eighth week of gestation
    D. the twenty-eighth and thirty-eighth week of gestation   (6:302)

127. Which of the following drugs, given to prevent premature labor, blocks sensitivity of the myometrium?
    A. vasodilan
    B. ethanol
    C. ethisterone
    D. none of the above   (6:303)

128. Which of the following women is *not* a good candidate for drug therapy aimed at stopping premature labor?
    A. the woman carrying a live infant
    B. the woman with intact membranes
    C. the woman with some evidence of cervical changes
    D. the woman with cervical dilatation of 4 cm or more   (6:303)

129. If labor is suspected in a patient heavily sedated for eclampsia, the nurse should
    A. omit all ordinary observations in order to avoid stimulation that might precipitate convulsions
    B. ignore previous precautions against stimulation since observations during labor are more important
    C. palpate the uterus and observe the perineum for show as on any other patient but with a minimum of stimulation
    D. give the woman nalorphine (Nalline) in order to avoid fetal distress   (4:473)

130. The first sign of excessive blood levels of magnesium sulfate is
    A. disappearance of knee-jerk reflex
    B. ringing in the ears
    C. cardiac arrhythmia
    D. respiratory depression   (8:206)

131. Which of the following fetal positions tends to produce a prolonged labor?
    A. ROA
    B. LOA
    C. ROP
    D. no difference among the three positions   (8:436—7)

132. Symptoms that indicate the laboring woman is hyperventilating are
    A. shortness of breath
    B. lowered blood pressure
    C. cramps in arms and legs
    D. numbness and tingling of fingers and toes   (6:301)

133. A transverse lie is frequently associated with
    A. diabetes
    B. placenta previa
    C. placenta abruptio
    D. toxemia   (6:307)

134. Transverse presentations are more likely to occur in which of the following?

    1. fetal anomalies
    2. multiple pregnancies
    3. multigravidas
    4. polyhydramnios

    A. 1, 2, 3
    B. 1, 4
    C. none of the above
    D. all of the above   (6:307)

135. The breech is considered to be fully engaged when

    A. the presenting part is visible at the vulva
    B. the buttocks are on the same plane as the ischial spines
    C. the buttocks are visible at the vulva
    D. none of the above   (6:309)

136. Usually, what is the first observed indication of a prolapsed cord?

    A. seeing the cord outside the vagina
    B. palpation of the cord below the PP on vaginal examination
    C. palpation of the cord beside the PP
    D. lowering of fetal heart rate (8:439—40)

137. Forceps were first used in obstetrical practice by

    A. Hugh Chamberlen
    B. Peter Chamberlen
    C. Palfyne
    D. Smellie   (8:449)

138. The most frequent indication for forceps is

    A. fetal complications
    B. maternal complications
    C. poor progress of fetal head
    D. none of the above   (8:450)

139. The delivery of the after-coming head is frequently facilitated by

    A. Simpson forceps
    B. Piper forceps
    C. Tarnier forceps
    D. Tucker-McLean forceps   (8:456)

140. The most common reason for a cesarean section is

    A. dystocia
    B. medical complications
    C. previous cesarean section
    D. bleeding   (8:458)

141. Which of the following is usually the preferred type of cesarean section?

    A. classical
    B. low cervical
    C. cesarean hysterectomy
    D. none of the above   (8:458)

142. Who was the first physician in the United States to perform a cesarean section?

    A. Max Sanger
    B. John Richmond
    C. Harold Mack
    D. none of the above   (6:330)

143. Who is given credit for originating the low cervical cesarean section?

    A. Joseph DeLee
    B. Douglas Haynes
    C. H. Sellheim
    D. none of the above   (6:330)

144. Postpartum hemorrhage following a cesarean section can be most accurately detected by

    A. palpating the fundus through the dressing
    B. removing the dressing and checking the fundus
    C. checking the perineal pads for amount of lochia
    D. checking the vital signs and amount of lochia on perineal pads   (8:461)

145. A patient undergoing oxytocin administration during labor should be carefully observed for which of the following?

    1. maternal blood pressure
    2. duration and consistency of contractions
    3. fetal heart rate and rhythm
    4. the degree of relaxation between contractions

    A. 1, 3
    B. 2, 4
    C. 1, 2, 3
    D. 1, 2, 3, 4   (8:445)

146. The transition area between the upper and lower segments of the uterus is called

    A. Braun's retraction ring
    B. Bandl's ring
    C. fundus
    D. none of the above   (6:242)

147. Retention of the placenta is caused by

    A. insufficient strength of uterine contractions

B. adhesions between the placenta and uterus
C. contraction of the uterus below the placenta
D. all of the above   (8:461)

148. Hypotonic uterine dysfunction most commonly occurs during the

A. latent phase
B. active phase
C. placental separation phase
D. immediate postpartum phase   (4:496)

149. A transverse arrest can occur as a result of an

A. attempt to correct a transverse lie
B. incorrect attitude of the fetal head in a breech position
C. incomplete rotation of the head in an occiput posterior position
D. attempt to perform a podalic version   (4:498)

150. Breech presentations occur in what percentage of all term deliveries?

A. 3%
B. 5%
C. 7%
D. 9%   (4:498)

151. The perinatal mortality rate of breech deliveries in the United States is about

A. 5%
B. 7%
C. 9%
D. 12%   (4:499)

152. Face presentations occur about

A. once in every 50 cases
B. once in every 100 cases
C. once in every 200 cases
D. once in every 300 cases   (4:501)

153. The infant mortality associated with large babies (over 4,500 g) has been estimated as

A. 10%
B. 13%
C. 20%
D. 25%   (4:502)

154. What congenital fetal abnormality is frequently encountered in breech deliveries?

A. hydrocephalus
B. anacephalus
C. Bell's palsy
D. club foot   (4:499)

155. Which of the following is given to control postpartum hemorrhage in which the cause is known to be hypofibrinogenemia?

A. parenogen
B. whole blood
C. dextran
D. pitocin   (6:317)

156. The most common cause of postpartum hemorrhage is

A. uterine atony
B. lacerations of the perineum
C. lacerations of the vagina
D. retained placental fragments   (4:504)

157. Which of the following actions would be carried out first in the treatment of excessive bleeding following separation of the placenta?

A. call the doctor
B. give an oxytocic
C. massage the uterus
D. prepare uterine packing   (4:505)

158. In which of the following cases would you *least* suspect uterine atony to occur?

A. birth of a premature baby
B. birth of twins weighing 5 lb each
C. birth of a 6-lb baby with presence of hydramnios
D. birth of a 7-lb baby under general anesthesia   (4:504)

159. The most common cause of a ruptured uterus is

A. prolonged labor in a multigravida
B. obstructed labor
C. rupture of a previous cesarean section scar
D. injudicious use of oxytocin in labor   (4:507)

160. Which of the following might indicate a laceration of the cervix or vaginal wall?

A. a firm, well-contracted uterus with no bleeding
B. a uterus that is boggy and a moderate amount of bleeding
C. a uterus that becomes firm following massage with decreased amount of bleeding
D. a uterus that is firm with excessive amount of bleeding   (8:462)

161. Hypofibrinogenemia occurs in 38% of what maternal complication?

    A. abruptio placentae
    B. placenta previa
    C. uterine atony
    D. none of the above   (6:198)

162. In a precipitate delivery the most important thing to do is

    A. provide a sterile field for the delivery of the infant
    B. provide equipment for the cutting of the cord
    C. prevent aspiration of fluids by the child
    D. wash hands to prevent infection (8:424)

163. When expelling the placenta from the vagina or lower uterine segment, pressure against a relaxed uterus may cause

    A. excessive bleeding
    B. increased relaxation of uterine muscle
    C. prolapse of uterine fundus
    D. none of the above   (8:414)

164. Which of the following pH readings obtained by a fetal capillary scalp blood sample would indicate that the fetus is in distress?

    A. 7.4
    B. 7.3
    C. 7.2
    D. 7.1   (6:321)

165. A multiparous patient should be transferred to the delivery room when

    A. she is 5 cm dilated
    B. she is 7 to 9 cm dilated
    C. there is bulging of the perineum
    D. the caput is visible   (3:455)

166. When a laboring woman is in the second stage of labor, ideally she should be transferred to the delivery room

    A. quickly, so as to avoid an unattended delivery in the bed
    B. quickly, because she may not be able to continue her breathing pattern on the moving bed
    C. unhurriedly, so as to give the doctor ample time to get ready for the delivery
    D. unhurriedly, because the rushed environment increases the woman's general anxiety   (3:465)

167. The incidence of twins in the white race is approximately

    A. once in every 50 cases
    B. once in every 100 cases
    C. once in every 150 cases
    D. once in every 175 cases   (4:510)

168. The main cause of uterine dysfunction is

    A. ill-timed and excessive administration of the analgesic
    B. minor degrees of pelvic contractions
    C. slight extension of fetal head
    D. overdistention of the uterus   (2:194)

169. During vaginal examinations the woman in labor should be

    A. free from interference by the father, who should be asked to leave
    B. encouraged to relax and breathe deeply in order to facilitate the examination
    C. placed in a modified Sim's position in order to prevent fecal-vaginal contamination
    D. encouraged to "pant" in order to retard the descent of the presenting part (8:369)

170. In many labor rooms, women lie flat on their backs during labor

    A. in order to facilitate nursing and medical care
    B. because this is always the most comfortable position
    C. in order to decrease the possibility of hypotensive syndrome
    D. because a sitting or side-lying position will interfere with the mechanism of labor   (8:338-63)

Directions: Each group of numbered words or phrases is followed by a list of lettered statements. MATCH the lettered statement with the numbered word or phrase most closely associated with it.

Questions 171 through 174

171. entrance of the presenting part into the superior pelvic strait
172. smallest anterior-posterior diameter of fetal head
173. greatest transverse of the fetal head
174. change of shape of the fetal head

    A. suboccipitobregmatic
    B. engagement
    C. molding
    D. biparietal   (8:260-1)

Questions 175 through 178
175. saddle block anesthesia
176. general anesthesia
177. self-administered anesthesia
178. regional anesthesia

    A. methoxyflurane
    B. Xylocaine
    C. Novocain with glucose
    D. cyclopropane   (8:317−23)

Questions 179 through 182
179. heart rate in the intervals between the various normal periodic fetal heart rate changes
180. heart rate slows briefly before acme and then returns to normal by end of contraction
181. heart rate slows after acme and then continues to decrease
182. heart rate in which the fetal heart may not rise much above 100 beats/min

    A. bradycardia
    B. basal heart rate
    C. lack of oxygen to fetus
    D. compression of fetal head   (8:353−6)

Directions: This part of the test consists of a situation followed by a series of incomplete statements. Study the situation and select the BEST answer to complete each statement that follows.

Questions 183 through 194
Ms. Janet Marsh, a 21-year-old gravida I, is admitted to the labor and delivery room unit in her thirty-ninth week of gestation. She is having uterine contractions occurring every five minutes and lasting about forty seconds each, of moderate intensity. She has intact membranes and has had a bloody show.

183. Ms. Marsh is probably in

    A. false labor
    B. early labor
    C. late active labor
    D. second stage of labor   (2:142)

184. Ms. Marsh's baby will probably be

    A. an immature infant
    B. a premature infant
    C. a term infant
    D. a postmature infant   (4:114)

Pelvic examination reveals a 2- to 3-cm dilatation with 80% effacement of the cervix. The vertex is presenting and is at a +1 station. Vital signs are within normal limits; the fetal heart rate is 144 beats/min and the heart beat is located in the lower left quadrant.

185. After the evaluation of Janet's labor and general health, the nurse palpates Janet's abdomen to determine

    A. presentation, descent, dilatation
    B. fetal movement, position, effacement
    C. fetal outline, presentation, attitude
    D. fetal position, presentation, engagement   (8:274)

186. On admission, the vertex was said to be at +1 station. This means that the head

    A. has just entered the true pelvis
    B. has just entered the false pelvis
    C. is just below the ischial spines
    D. will proceed no further   (8:273)

187. It is learned from the abdominal and pelvic examination that the baby's back is toward Ms. Marsh's left and slightly anterior, and the head is well flexed and cannot be dislodged from the pelvic inlet. These observations would be recorded as

    A. LOP engaged
    B. LOA engaged
    C. LOP floating
    D. ROA engaged   (8:268−9, 273)

188. Ms. Marsh's labor causes slow but continuous change in the cervix. Four hours after admission, the end of the first phase of labor becomes evident. Which of the following indicates that she is moving into the second phase of labor?

    A. an uncontrollable desire to push
    B. sudden calmness and relaxation
    C. the shortening of duration and stronger intensity of the contractions
    D. apprehension and social withdrawal increased   (2:142; 8:295)

189. About four hours later, Janet appears tense during and following contractions, and even with much support from her husband, cannot relax. The doctor is notified and orders Demerol 50 mg and Phenergan 50 mg. This combination of medication will produce

    A. a twilight sleep in Ms. Marsh
    B. relaxation by elevating Ms. Marsh's pain threshold
    C. relaxation by decreasing Ms. Marsh's pain threshold
    D. little relief, since it is a small dose   (8:314−5)

190. Nine hours after admission, Ms. Marsh expresses the desire to push with her contractions. Her husband, who has been

with her fairly constantly, seems confused and upset about Janet's inability to follow the deep breathing pattern he has been encouraging thus far in labor. The nurse would be most helpful to Mr. and Ms. Marsh if she intervened by

A. telling Mr. Marsh to take a half-hour lunch break and promising to stay with his wife while he is gone
B. calling Mr. Marsh away from the labor room and explaining to him how he should encourage his wife to push
C. explaining the method of breathing, holding, and bearing down to Mr. and Mrs. Marsh during the next contraction
D. between the next contraction explaining to both Mr. and Ms. Marsh how Ms. Marsh should push and help her practice once.   (8:340)

191. After 30 minutes of pushing, when the fetal head is crowning, Ms. Marsh is moved to the delivery room. The physician administers local anesthesia into the perineum, then performs a midline episiotomy. The leading disadvantage of the midline over the mediolateral site for an episotomy is

A. slowness of healing causes prolonged discomfort
B. the possibility of tearing through a sphincter muscle
C. scar tissue causing limited perineal stretching for the next delivery
D. greater blood loss   (8:387–8)

192. Baby girl Marsh is born in the next several minutes. Her cry is spontaneous, and breathing is established within 30 seconds. Her apgar rating will probably be

A. 10
B. 9
C. 8
D. 7
E. 6   (8:392–3)

193. Ten minutes after the delivery of the infant baby girl, the placenta is delivered with the smooth fetal surface outermost. This mechanism of expulsion of the placenta is called

A. Crede's method
B. Schultze's method
C. cotyledon
D. Duncan's method   (2:133)

194. Which of the following drugs would probably be given to Ms. Marsh for the purpose of providing strong and prolonged uterine contractions with little likelihood of elevation of blood pressure?

A. Ergotrate
B. Pitocin
C. Syntocinon
D. Methergine   (4:336)

Questions 195 through 200
Ms. Jane Clemmons, a 28-year-old gravida II, para I, at about 36 weeks of gestation notifies her doctor that she is "bleeding" and is experiencing "abdominal cramps." He recommends that she report to the labor and delivery room at once, then notifies the nursing staff to call him when she arrives. You are the nurse in charge.

195. At this time which of the following applies to Ms. Clemmons?

A. she is in premature labor
B. she has placenta previa
C. she has placenta abruptio
D. not able to tell at this time   (4:480–2)

196. Which of the following is of greatest importance for you to find out about Ms. Clemmons?

A. length of previous labor
B. amount of bleeding
C. size of last baby
D. last menstrual period   (4:481)

197. Which of the following routine admission procedures would be omitted for Ms. Clemmons?

A. taking of vital signs
B. listening to fetal heart
C. vaginal or rectal exam
D. routine blood work   (4:481)

Ms. Clemmons arrives within fifteen minutes. She reports that she is now having contractions every five minutes lasting about forty seconds and has saturated one perineal pad since leaving home. Her vital signs are within normal limits; fetal heart sounds are 144 and located in the lower right quadrant. The abdomen is soft between contractions, and abdominal palpation reveals an ROA with floating presenting part.

198. The doctor arrives and makes a tentative diagnosis of

A. placenta previa
B. abruptio placentae with concealed hemorrhage

C. normal labor
D. none of the above   (8:192—8)

199. The doctor then decides to do a "double set up" examination. This means that he will
A. do a rectal examination, and if there is no bleeding, he will do a vaginal examination
B. do a vaginal examination followed by stimulation of labor and delivery by forceps if necessary
C. do a vaginal examination with equipment ready to do an immediate cesarean section if necessary
D. none of the above   (4:481)

200. At the time of the vaginal examination, the doctor finds that Ms. Clemmons has a partial placenta previa. He decides to
A. allow the woman to labor normally
B. stimulate labor to move more quickly
C. plan on forceps delivery to hasten the second stage of labor
D. do a cesarean section   (4:481)

Questions 201 through 211
Ms. Sarah Johnston, gravida 2, para 0, is a 22-year-old woman who is admitted to the labor and delivery unit for an induction. According to her last menstrual period, she is 18 days over her estimated date of confinement. An initial vaginal examination reveals that her cervix is a fingertip dilated and there is 50% effacement.

201. The fact that Ms. Johnston is a gravida 2, para 0 indicates that
A. she has been pregnant twice and has one living child
B. she has been pregnant twice and delivered a stillborn infant
C. she has been pregnant twice and her first pregnancy terminated in a nonviable fetus
D. none of the above   (8:136)

202. If Ms. Johnston's EDC has been calculated correctly, which of the following tentative diagnoses can be made regarding her infant?
A. the child may be a postmature infant
B. the child will be a victim of placental dysfunction
C. both A and B
D. neither A nor B   (6:440)

203. Ms. Johnston has been admitted for the purpose of induction of labor. This means that
A. the pregnancy will be terminated by surgical intervention in the form of a cesarean section
B. the labor will be artificially brought in after the fetus has reached a period of viability
C. Ms. Johnston will be carefully observed for 24 hours to determine her present condition and to watch for signs of labor
D. none of the above   (4:456)

204. Which of the following are classified as procedures for induction of labor?
1. use of castor oil
2. high, hot soapsuds enema
3. intravenous drip of oxytocin in a glucose and water solution
4. amniotomy
5. quinine sulfate
A. 1, 3, 4, 5
B. 2, 3, 4
C. 3, 4
D. all of the above   (4:456—8; 6:327—8)

205. Which of the following should be present in Ms. Johnston if the induction is to be successful?
1. cervix soft and partially effaced
2. cervix at least 1.5 cm dilated
3. regular uterine contractions coming at least every five minutes
4. fetal head fixed in the pelvis
A. 1, 4
B. 1, 2, 3
C. 1, 2, 4
D. all of the above   (8:443)

206. The doctor performs an amniotomy on Ms. Johnston. The first thing the nurse should do following this procedure is
A. check the blood pressure
B. check the fetal heart sounds
C. check the sheet and pad on which the woman is lying
D. check the pulse   (8:443)

207. Which of the following tests done during pregnancy would indicate that Ms. Johnston's baby was postmature?
A. serial estriol level
B. amniotic fluid analysis
C. both A and B
D. neither A nor B   (6:95)

208. Following the amniotomy, the physician starts an intravenous drip of 5% glucose and water with Pitocin added to it. You should observe Ms. Johnston carefully for

A. change in fetal heart sounds
B. tetanic contractions
C. rise or fall in blood pressure
D. all of the above (8:435)

209. The fetal heart rate should be checked at least

A. every 5 minutes
B. every 10 minutes
C. every 15 minutes
D. every 30 minutes (8:445)

210. After six hours of oxytocin therapy, Ms. Johnston is having mild contractions and her cervix is 1 to 2 cm dilated. There is slightly more effacement than was present on the previous examination. Which of the following statements is most accurate in indicating Ms. Johnston's present status in labor?

A. latent phase of cervical dilatation
B. active phase of cervical dilatation
C. acceleration phase
D. none of the above (8:295)

211. After 10 hours of oxytocic treatment, Ms. Johnston's cervix is 2 to 3 cm dilated. The physician decides to discontinue the intravenous drip and perform a cesarean section. He will probably do a

A. classical
B. low cervical
C. cesarean hysterectomy
D. none of the above (8:458)

Questions 212 through 215
Mrs. Ruth Smith is admitted to the labor and delivery unit. She is having 3- to 4-minute strong contractions lasting 55 to 60 seconds. She has a good bloody show, and membranes are intact. On rectal examination, the cervix is 4 to 5 cm dilated and 50% effaced. An hour after admission, Mrs. Smith suddenly experiences sharp abdominal pain and cries out for help. As you check the fundus you find it hard and board-like, and there is no increase in vaginal bleeding.

212. Mrs. Smith's symptoms are suggestive of

A. possible imminent delivery
B. possible placenta previa
C. possible abruptio placentae
D. possible cord prolapse (8:197–8)

213. You quickly check her pulse, which has increased in rate from 86 to 120, yet her blood pressure remains stable. This would indicate

A. beginning infection
B. beginning of second stage
C. beginning sign of hemorrhage
D. beginning of third stage (4:482)

214. Placenta previa indicates

A. separation of a normally implanted placenta
B. low implantation of the placenta
C. placenta will be delivered before labor starts
D. the placenta is malformed (4:480)

215. Absolute bed rest was ordered to

A. prevent premature labor
B. prevent further bleeding
C. lower metabolism because of bleeding
D. prevent toxemia (2:117)

Answers and Explanations:
Intrapartal Period

1. **D.** The uterine stretch theory holds that any hollow organ tends to contract and empty itself when distended to a certain point. Believers in the oxytocin theory indicate that higher blood levels of this hormone initiate labor by increasing the sensitivity of the uterus to the stimulating effect of the hormone. In the progesterone deprivation theory, it is believed that the lowering of the progesterone level upsets the balance between estrogen and progesterone, and labor results.

2. **B.** The fetal heart rate may change during and immediately following a contraction.

3. **A.** The mechanism of labor is defined as "the sequence of passive movements of the presenting part that permits passage through the birth canal."

4. **D.** The fetus expels the meconium into the amniotic fluid, giving the fluid a yellowish-green or dark green color.

5. **C.** Cervical effacement is one of the major changes that takes place during the first stage of labor.

6. **D.** This is caused by the shoulders of the baby undergoing a rotation to the anterior-posterior position corresponding to the rotation of the head.

7. **D.** Labor may deplete the woman's glycogen reserve. Usually during this period, intravenous dextrose solution and regular insulin are given.

8. **A.** Demerol (meperidine hydrochloride) resembles morphine as an analgesic; however, it is believed to be less of a respiratory depressant than morphine.

9. **A.** Forceps operations are usually designated as low when the fetal head has reached the perineal floor, has rotated into the anterior-posterior position, and the head is visible.

10. **A.** Correct recognition of both the fontanels and the sutures will determine the fetal position.

11. **C.** Narcotic drugs are not usually given until labor has been well established and when the delivery is not anticipated within two hours.

12. **B.** The ischial spines are felt on the side walls of the pelvis. An imaginary line is drawn between the two spines, then the vertical distance between this imaginary line and the lowest portion of the presenting part is estimated in centimeters.

13. **C.** A complete breech is also called full breech presentation.

14. **D.** One of the purposes of Braxton Hicks contractions is to begin effacement of the cervix.

15. **D.** Sparteine sulfate, when used as recommended, produces a gradual onset of regular contractions similar to those observed during a normal labor. Ruptured uteri have been reported following the use of this drug.

16. **A.** Ergotrate 0.18 mg is given orally three to four times daily.

17. **B.** When postpartum bleeding reaches 500 mL or more, the term postpartum hemorrhage is used.

18. **D.** If the presenting part is not engaged, there is the possibility of a prolapsed cord.

19. **A.** This stage starts with the onset of regular contractions and ends with full dilatation of the cervix.

20. **D.** Fourteen hours is an average figure. Some labors will be shorter, others much longer.

21. **B.** The second stage of the multigravida labor averages 30 minutes, whereas, in the primipara, the second stage equals 80 minutes.

22. **D.** The doctor will also observe changes in the cervix.

23. **A.** Lightening is the sensation of decreased abdominal distention produced by the descent of the uterus into the pelvic cavity.

24. **B.** The Braxton Hicks contractions may become painful in the last weeks of pregnancy and be interpreted as true labor pains.

25. **B.** As the cervix becomes ready for labor, it shortens and the canal enlarges, expelling the mucous plug. The supervical mucosa from the canal is expelled with the plug, thus causing the bloody show.

26. **A.** False labor contractions are the Braxton Hicks contractions that have become uncomfortable.

27. **B.** The increased intrauterine pressure makes these contractions uncomfortable for the woman.

28. **D.** During the increment phase the intensity of the contraction increases. This phase is also known as the crescendo phase.

29. **D.** The primigravida may do better if she stays at home until her contractions are five to eight minutes apart, providing there are not complications and she does not live a great distance from the hospital.

30. **B.** It is difficult to determine the exact time of onset of labor for a variety of reasons.

31. **A.** If labor does not occur within this time, and if the fetus is mature enough for extrauterine life, labor will probably be induced.

32. **C.** Sometimes particles of vernix caseosa can be seen in the fluid.

33. **B.** As labor progresses, the contractions increase in intensity and frequency until they recur every 3 to 4 minutes and increase in length until each contraction lasts from 50 to 75 seconds or longer.

34. **D.** The measurement of intrauterine pressure gives accurate information about the strength of uterine contractions that can not be obtained by usual clinical observations.

35. **C.** The Nitrazine test determines the presence or absence of amniotic fluid in the vagina. When the color change on the Nitrazine paper indicates that the pH of the vaginal section being tested is 7 or above, it is assumed that the membranes are ruptured.

36. **D.** The cervix enlarges to an average diameter of 10 cm.

37. **A.** The cervix of the multigravida at the onset of labor is about 2 cm dilated.

38. **A.** The multigravidas are often fully effaced before labor starts.

39. **C.** This phase is so named because of the rapid changes that are taking place in the body at this time.

40. **B.** During this latent phase, contractions also become well established, and the cervix may dilate several centimeters.

41. **C.** The oozing may increase suddenly as the dilatation becomes complete.

42. **B.** During the active phase, cervical dilatation progresses rapidly.

43. **B.** This stage begins with complete dilatation of the cervix and ends with complete delivery of the infant.

44. **C.** Combined efforts of the uterine muscle and abdominal muscle contractions are most effective in the expulsion of the infant.

45. **C.** Following crowning, the infant's head no longer recedes between contractions. Birth of the infant is imminent.

46. **A.** During placental separation, the uterus becomes a globular shape.

47. **C.** In the Schultz mechanism, the shiny fetal surface presents at the vaginal outlet first.

48. **D.** All of the terms are used to describe the labor period.

49. **D.** This is the shortest but most uncomfortable period for the woman.

50. **A.** During this time, the contractions last longer, are more frequent and stronger. Rupture of the membranes may occur at this time.

51. **B.** The most common attitude is one of complete flexion in which the fetus' chin touches its chest, arms are folded across chest, and legs are flexed into the abdomen.

52. **B.** This is a critical period for the mother, and one in which the vital signs should stabilize and any tendency for immediate hemorrhage should be controlled.

53. **B.** The cervix at this time may be described as "very pliable" or "butter soft."

54. **B.** The largest diameter has now passed the ischial spine, another possible obstacle during the birth process.

55. **C.** Intravenous oxytocic drip, with or without concomitant artificial amniotomy, is the most frequently used method of induction at term.

56. **C.** This type of utermine contraction pattern may be indicative of impending tonic uterine contraction.

57. **D.** Electrocardiographic tracings of the fetal heart indicate that it has several different kinds of normal variation in rate. The baseline upon which all of these variations in rate are superimposed is the basal fetal heart rate.

58. **C.** The basal rate for each fetus normally remains constant with a variation of 4 to 6 beats/min.

59. **D.** The normal, rapid baseline fluctuations are rarely heard with intermediate stethoscopic monitoring.

60. **C.** A slowing of the fetal heart during a contraction is not normal with the exception of some brief types that cannot be picked up with or are not usually detected with a stethoscope.

61. **C.** Continuous monitoring is more accurate in terms of detecting fetal distress than is the intermediate fetoscopic monitoring, because it is possible to determine relationships between contractions and fetal heart patterns.

62. **B.** Constant positioning on the back puts the weight of the baby on the large abdominal blood vessels and interferes with the return of blood from the lower extremities.

63. **A.** Demerol is usually given intramuscularly in a dose of 50 to 100 mg.

64. **C.** A narcotic is given at least two hours prior to delivery to avoid its effect on the baby.

65. **A.** They are most useful in decreasing apprehension during early labor. The usual dose is 100 to 300 mg orally, intramuscularly, or intravenously.

66. **B.** Scopolamine without adequate analgesia produces excitement, hallucinations, and delirium.

67. **A.** A local infiltration is used for performing and repairing episiotomies and repairing lacerations, which is all that is minimally necessary for the prepared woman.

68. **B.** The nerves that supply the uterus, vagina, bladder, and rectum are distributed in the pelvic plexus.

69. **B.** There is relief of pain from the uterine contractions and dilatation of the cervix.

70. **C.** An epidural can be given once the woman is in active labor. If given correctly, the epidural does not inhibit uterine contractions.

71. **A.** Accidental injection of the local anesthetic solution into the subarachnoid space will produce spinal anesthesia and the resulting difficulty in movement of the legs.

72. **B.** There is a cumulative effect of Pentrane in the body, and the nurse should be ready to reduce the dosage should side effects appear. Also, slow and shallow respirations indicate a need to reduce the dosage.

73. **D.** The anesthesia of choice is a local infiltration or a pudendal block with intermittent nitrous oxide. The woman is thus able to push the breech out herself. If difficulty arises during the delivery of shoulders or head, cyclopropane or halothane can be used.

74. **B.** The hypotension is the result of sympathetic block and is usually related to the level of anesthesia obtained.

75. **C.** Sir James Simpson of Scotland first used ether anesthesia in obstetrical practice during the year 1847.

76. **A.** The occiput is used in defining fetal position.

77. **D.** The nurse best evaluates the contractions by placing her hand on the fundus of the uterus and leaving it there through several contractions.

78. **C.** The intensity of the contraction can be felt by noting the tautness of the abdominal wall. As an example, at the peak of a contraction if the consistency of the fundal portion is similar to the firmness of the bony area of the forehead, it is a strong contraction.

79. **C.** The uterine souffle is produced by blood rushing through the large vessels of the uterus and is the same as the maternal pulse.

80. **C.** Statistics indicate that the woman laboring with a breech presentation does not have a harder labor than any other laboring woman.

81. **D.** There is a possibility of a prolapsed cord if the presenting part is not down and against the cervix.

82. **D.** This position may assist in the normal anterior rotation of the vertex to the anterior position.

83. **B.** Cramping of the legs at this time occurs because of pressure, and the nurse should make every attempt to lessen this discomfort.

84. **C.** This is behavior characteristic of the transitional phase. The woman needs to have someone with her and be told that she is doing very well. She does not, however, want to be bothered.

85. **C.** The woman should be informed that the wrist cuffs are used to prevent injury.

86. **C.** The woman is very introverted at this time. The nurse may have to repeat instructions before the woman understands what is happening.

87. **D.** This can be very uncomfortable for the woman. Both legs are also lowered at the same time for the same reason.

88. **B.** The parents, particularly the woman, see childbirth as the end of a long nine-month waiting period, rather than the beginning of a new life.

89. **D.** The nursing care remains flexible and is based on the needs of each individual, woman, husband, and infant.

90. **C.** The vital signs are taken every four hours unless there is a fever present in the woman or there has been prolonged labor. Then the vital signs may be repeated every two hours or sometimes more often.

91. **D.** The need for physical contact will vary from patient to patient. The woman herself will usually indicate the kind and amount of contact she wants and from whom she wants it.

92. **D.** The perineal shave serves a purpose both during the delivery and in the postpartum period. The partial prep (perineum only) is becoming increasingly popular and is of less discomfort to the woman than the total skin preparation (symphysis pubis and perineum).

93. **D.** A full stomach during labor may cause discomfort to the woman and create problems of aspiration of vomitus if the woman receives a general anesthetic.

94. **C.** An enema may stimulate uterine contractions and cause more bleeding.

95. **C.** Pain in the lower back may cause more discomfort than the abdominal pain caused by uterine contractions. The massage may be done by either nurse or husband.

96. **C.** It helps if the mother is assisted to do pant-blow breathing during a contraction as a means of reducing the urge to push down. Backache may be due to fetal position, weight of uterus pressing on the spinal cord, or lying in one position for a long period of time.

97. **B.** If a headache develops, the blood pressure should be checked. Then the nurse should check with the doctor regarding her observations.

98. **C.** At times it is difficult to determine the difference between a bloody show and vaginal bleeding. If in question, the nurse should check with the doctor.

99. **C.** A tear that extends up the anterior wall of the rectum is sometimes termed a fourth-degree laceration.

100. **C.** If the cord is around the infant's neck, the doctor will either clamp the cord and cut at once or slip the cord over the head.

101. **D.** It is important that the nurse show acceptance of the woman's behavior at this time.

102. **B.** The contractions at this time will be coming about every 2 to 4 minutes, lasting 45 to 90 seconds.

103. **C.** This type of uterine contraction pattern should be reported to the doctor at once. It can result in ruptured uterus for mother and asphyxia in the infant.

104. **A.** Conscious release of muscles during and between contractions is also begun.

105. **A.** The occiput emerges from under the pubic arch. Extension becomes complete when the infant's head is born.

106. **B.** The resistance of the pelvic floor pushes the fetal head forward and toward the vaginal opening, thus bringing about extension.

107. **B.** Ritgen maneuver is performed between contractions. As the head crowns, the doctor exerts pressure through the perineum on the infant's chin. Using the other hand, he exerts pressure on the occiput. This controls the delivery of the head.

108. **A.** Panting reduces involuntary bearing down and the resultant intra-abdominal pressure. This in turn helps to prevent rapid advancement of the head.

109. **A.** The mother should see her newborn infant as soon as possible, as there is a mounting anxiety about the child's condition if the interval between its birth and seeing it is prolonged.

110. **D.** The chills may be caused by emotional or physiological factors, or an interaction of the two.

111. **C.** This method of removal of the placenta is called the Brandt-Andrews' maneuver.

112. **C.** If the membranes are ruptured, the pH in the vaginal canal will be 6.5 to 7.5.

113. **B.** In the internal system of fetal monitoring, fetal heart rate and uterine contractions can be recorded simultaneously.

114. **C.** The term "pain" has always been associated with the uterine contractions of childbirth, and many women still approach childbirth with a fear of pain.

115. **C.** The normal blood fibrinogen level during pregnancy is 250 to 500 mg/dL.

116. **D.** All of the points mentioned are considered to be advantages of delivering in a recumbent position.

117. **C.** Three factors are involved in the process of labor —powers, passenger, and passage. Thus, dystocia may be caused by deviation from normal in any one of these three factors.

118. **C.** Excessive or too early administration of analgesia causes uterine dysfunction.

119. **D.** Labor may be prolonged or arrested in any one of the cervical dilation phases or in the fetal descent period.

120. **D.** Large size of infants has been found to be significantly related to dysfunctional labor.

121. **B.** In hypertonic uterine dysfunction, the contractions are very painful but ineffectual in producing anything more than minor progress in the labor.

122. **B.** Morphine 1/4 g may be given to ease contractions. A short-acting barbiturate may be given to provide rest, as normal labor usually starts after a period of rest.

123. **C.** Elevation of the vital signs heralds the onset of secondary complications.

124. **A.** By definition, a precipitous labor and delivery is three hours or less in duration.

125. **C.** Premature rupture also occurs more frequently with hydramnios and fetopelvic disproportion.

126. **D.** A premature labor is one that occurs between the twenty-eighth and thirty-eighth week of gestation.

127. **C.** Pregneninolone sulfate (ethisterone), 5 mg per minute in 5% dextrose solution, blocks sensitivity of the myometrium.

128. **D.** Other factors that make the woman a poor candidate for drug therapy are ruptured membranes and evidence of infection or bleeding.

129. **C.** Labor in eclampsia may proceed with few external signs. Thus the nurse must palpate the uterus and watch the perineum.

130. **A.** The knee-jerk reflex disappears before respiratory depression occurs.

131. **C.** The occiput in the posterior position must rotate a longer distance to reach the symphysis pubis than the occiput in the anterior position. This prolongs the second stage of labor.

132. **D.** Panting forces carbon dioxide from the woman's lungs. The blood becomes alkaline because of the depletion of carbon dioxide. Symptoms also include dizziness and vomiting.

133. **B.** The placenta previa prohibits the engagement of the presenting part.

134. **D.** Transverse presentations are more likely to occur in all the conditions mentioned in the question.

135. **C.** The breech is considered fully engaged when the buttocks are visible at the vulva, indicating ample room for the head.

136. **D.** The slowing of the fetal heart is due to cord compression.

137. **B.** Although Peter Chamberlen and members of his family started using the forceps early in the seventeenth century, knowledge about the instrument was not shared with other physicians until the beginning of the eighteenth century.

138. **C.** Slow progress of the fetal head may be due to poor uterine and abdominal muscles, great resistance of the perineal muscles, or failure of the head to rotate.

139. **B.** The Piper forceps are particularly designed to fit the after-coming head.

140. **C.** The most common cause for the primary cesarean section is dystocia, usually caused by cephalopelvic disproportion.

141. **B.** The low segment cesarean section is considered the preferred procedure because there is a decreased danger of infection and a decreased probability of uterine rupture in subsequent pregnancies.

142. **B.** John Lambert Richmond performed the first cesarean section in the United States on April 22, 1827.

143. **C.** H. Sellheim originated the low cervical cesarean section in 1908.

144. **D.** Checking the blood pressure, pulse rate, and amount of lochia should give a fairly good estimate of the degree of intrauterine bleeding.

145. **D.** The woman who is undergoing oxytocin administration should have her blood pressure and fetal heart tones checked every 15 minutes, and there should be constant evaluation of the uterine contraction-relaxation pattern.

146. **A.** Braun's retraction ring is a normal physiologic retraction ring. In obstructed labors this ring may become more pronounced and is then known as Bandl's ring.

147. **D.** A retained placenta is one that is not expelled within half an hour following delivery of the infant. All of the factors stated can contribute to the retention of the placenta within the uterus.

148. **B.** Hypotonic uterine dysfunction occurs during the accelerated or active phase, or during the second stage.

149. **C.** The transverse arrest is a deviation from the normal mechanism of labor and may adversely affect uterine behavior.

150. **A.** Breech presentations occur in about 3% of all term deliveries.

151. **D.** Breech deliveries are considered thus to be complicated labors, and an obstetrician should be available for immediate medical assistance.

152. **C.** The face presentation usually terminates spontaneously with the chin in the anterior position.

153. **B.** The high mortality rate is due to the trauma associated with the delivery process.

154. **A.** Hydrocephalus is seen in about one third of all breech deliveries. The enlarged cranium is too large to fit into the pelvic inlet.

155. **A.** Parenogen 4 to 10 g is given intravenously.

156. **A.** The uterine muscles fail to contract because of fatigue of the muscles themselves.

157. **C.** Massage of the uterus will stimulate the muscles to contract, thus controlling the blood loss.

158. **A.** Overdistention of the uterus is one of the major causes of hemorrhage.

159. **C.** The most frequent time for rupture is during the laboring process. However, the rupture can also occur in pregnancy.

160. **D.** If a laceration is present, the bleeding is controlled by approximating the lacerated edges of the cervix or vaginal walls with sutures.

161. **A.** Hypofibrinogenemia occurs in approximately 10 to 38% of abruptio placentae cases.

162. **C.** Immediately following birth, the child should be held with its head lower than the rest of the body so that fluids can drain from the air passages.

163. **C.** Pressure against a relaxed uterus can cause inversion of the uterus and the prolapse of the uterine fundus.

164. **D.** A pH value below 7.2 in the fetus indicates that the fetus is in distress.

165. **B.** The multiparous patient should be transferred during the transition period (7−9 cm) to avoid the last-minute frenzy which causes tension for all of those involved.

166. **D.** The frantic activity involved in last-minute rushes to the delivery room adds to the general uneasiness of the woman and also to the anxiety of the husband.

167. **B.** They occur about once in every 73 births in the nonwhite races.

168. **A.** The drugs are given too early in the labor or too much is given at any one time.

169. **B.** The vaginal examination causes additional stress to the laboring woman, and every attempt should be made to make the woman as comfortable as possible.

170. **A.** During labor the woman is usually requested to be flat on her back for the checking of cervical dilatation and fetal heart tones. This position can result in hypotensive syndrome. Usually, the woman can remain in the position most comfortable for her.

171. **B.** Engagement means that the presenting part has entered into the superior pelvic strait (inlet of the pelvis).

172. **A.** The suboccipitobregmatic diameter is measured from the undersurface of the occiput to the center of the anterior fontanel and is 9.5 cm.

173. **D.** The biparietal diameter is the greatest transverse diameter and is the distance between the parietal protuberances. It measures 9.25 cm.

174. **C.** In molding, opposing margins of bones meet, or overlap to such a degree that the shape of the head changes and certain diameters are appreciably diminished.

175. **C.** The addition of glucose to an agent used for regional anesthesia makes the agent heavy and facilitates its localization.

176. **D.** Cyclopropane is used for continuous pain relief rather than intermittent pain relief because of its explosive nature, which makes frequent removal of the mask a potential explosion hazard.

177. **A.** Methoxyflurane (Pentrane) may also be used as an inhalation anesthetic agent during the latter part of the first stage and during the second stage. Toxic side effects include maternal hypotension and infant respiratory depression.

178. **B.** Both a local and pudendal nerve block can be done by the infiltration of Xylocaine.

179. **B.** The normal basal fetal heart rate is between 125 and 155 beats/min, although in the majority of infants, the rate is between 130 and 140 beats/min.

180. **D.** This heart rate is characteristic of type I dips. The compression of the fetal head during contractions results in stimulation of the vagus nerve and a transient rise in the vagal tone, which in turn slows the heart rate.

181. **C.** This heart rate is characteristic of type II dips, and is a sign of fetal hypoxia.

182. **A.** Persistent bradycardia may occur if the cause of fetal distress is not found and taken care of.

183. **B.** The onset of regular uterine contractions is considered by many to be the onset of labor. Contractions coming about every 5 minutes lasting about 40 seconds each indicate early labor.

184. **C.** The average duration from the time of conception is 38 weeks or 266 days. Calculating from the first day of the last menstrual period, the average length of pregnancy is 40 weeks or 280 days. However, by definition, a premature infant is an infant born prior the thirty-seventh week of gestation. Thus, a pregnancy terminating at the thirty-ninth week of gestation can be considered at term.

185. **D.** Palpation is probably the most useful method for determining the presentation, position, and degree of engagement during the latter months of pregnancy and during labor.

186. **C.** When the presenting part is at the level of the ischial spines, it is at 0 station. As it descends lower into the birth canal, it becomes +1, +2, etc.

187. **B.** The letters LOA indicate left occiput anterior. Engagement indicates that the biparietal plane (of the head) has passed through the pelvic inlet.

188. **D.** The second phase of labor (active phase) occurs when the cervix becomes about 4 cm dilated.

189. **B.** The Demerol provides considerable relief from the discomfort but does not completely eliminate the pain. Phenergan enhances the action of the Demerol.

190. **D.** Mr. Marsh should be included and supported in his attempts to help his wife. Ms. Marsh will be more able to listen if explanations are made clear during the less stressful periods of her labor.

191. **B.** The advantages of a midline incision are that it is easier to repair and it heals well, which will allow far less discomfort.

192. **A.** An infant in excellent condition at birth can receive the highest score possible—that of 10.

193. **B.** The Schultze method is the most common method of placental delivery.

194. **D.** Methergine, a semisynthetic derivative of ergonovine, produces stronger and longer contractions than ergonovine and is less likely to produce high blood pressure. Pitocin (Syntocinon) produces strong contractions for 5 to 10 minutes, then normal rhythmic contractions return.

195. **D.** Further clarification of the "bleeding" and "abdominal cramps" is necessary before any of the other statements can apply.

196. **B.** Ms. Clemmons may have reported "bleeding" when in reality she is having a normal show.

197. **C.** The vaginal exam would not be done because digital examination of the cervix might precipitate increased bleeding.

198. **A.** In placenta previa, there is painless bleeding occurring during the later months of pregnancy. In abruptio placentae with concealed hemorrhage, there is pain associated with the bleeding and shock out of proportion to the amount of evident bleeding.

199. **C.** Digital examination of the cervix can precipitate increased bleeding, and cesarean section must be done at once.

200. **D.** In all cases of partial placenta previa, cesarean section is the method of choice for delivery.

201. **C.** Para refers to past pregnancies that continued to the period of viability.

202. **A.** A postmature infant is one who is live born after forty-two weeks' gestation.

203. **B.** An induction of labor is one in which there is an artificial bringing on of labor after the period of viability.

204. **D.** All of the mentioned are classified as procedures for induction of labor.

205. **C.** The cervix should show some of the changes that take place shortly before labor, and the head should be well down in the pelvis.

206. **B.** Following the rupture of the membranes, there is a chance that the cord will prolapse.

207. **C.** A decrease in serial estriol levels is present after the fortieth week of pregnancy. Analysis of the amniotic fluid provides information on postmaturity.

208. **D.** A tetanic contraction is one in which the uterus stays contracted continuously rather than relaxing at regular intervals. These contractions can produce interference with the placenta, causing asphyxia in the baby.

209. **C.** The fetal heart should be checked every 15 minutes or more often if indicated.

210. **A.** During the latent phase, contractions become established, effacement of the cervix takes place, and the cervix dilates to between 2 and 3 cm.

211. **B.** The low cervical cesarean section is usually the surgical procedure of choice. The possibility of postpartum infection is decreased, and there is less chance of rupture of the scar in subsequent pregnancies.

212. **C.** Mrs. Smith's symptoms are suggestive of abruptio placentae with a concealed hemorrhage.

213. **C.** Hemorrhage-induced shock is manifested by a rapid pulse.

214. **B.** In placenta previa, the placenta is attached to the lower uterine segment and either totally or partially covers the region of the cervix.

215. **B.** She should be kept quiet so that further bleeding is not activated.

CHAPTER 6

Postpartum Period

Following the birth of a child, the mother must make major adjustments in her own life style. These adjustments are made in relation to the members of her family, including the new member of the family whom she has nurtured for the past nine months.

Included in this chapter are questions relating to the normal recovery phases of the woman and the complications that can arise as a result of the childbearing experience.

The situational questions found at the end of this chapter examine both the normal and abnormal recovery periods.

The postpartum period is an ideal time to reinforce basic nursing skills and learn to perfect teaching skills. Since the environment on a postpartum unit is usually an unrushed one, there is ample opportunity to put into practice what has been learned.

Directions: Each of the questions or incomplete statements below is followed by four suggested answers or completions. Select the BEST answer in each case.

1. The term puerperium refers to
   A. return of body functioning following birth of the infant
   B. return of reproductive organs to their normal condition following delivery of the infant
   C. period between the delivery of the infant and discharge of mother and infant from the hospital
   D. the first four weeks post partum (4:359)

2. The process by which the uterus returns to a prepregnant state is achieved by
   A. involution
   B. subinvolution
   C. suprainvolution
   D. deinvolution (4:360)

3. The process by which the uterus returns to a prepregnant state starts
   A. immediately following delivery
   B. after the first 48 hours
   C. somewhere during the end of the first week
   D. about one day following birth of the infant (4:359)

4. About how much does the uterus weigh immediately following delivery?
   A. ½ lb
   B. ¾ lb
   C. 1 lb
   D. 2 lb (4:360)

5. Immediately after the delivery, the fundus is usually located
   A. directly above the umbilicus
   B. at the level of the umbilicus
   C. midway between symphysis pubis and umbilicus
   D. below the symphysis pubis (4:360)

6. The true level of the fundus cannot be determined if
   A. the woman has just eaten a large meal
   B. the woman has not had a good bowel movement
   C. the woman has a full bladder
   D. the woman has delivered a premature infant   (4:360)

7. When recording the height of the fundus during the postpartum period, which of the following measurements is most commonly used?
   A. centimeters
   B. inches
   C. finger breadths
   D. none of the above   (5:155)

8. When the mother complains about "after pains" this usually indicates that
   A. the mother is asking for extra attention
   B. the mother is still psychologically experienceing the labor
   C. the uterus is not contracting well
   D. the uterus is contracting normally for this period of time   (4:362)

9. Which decidual layer is shed during the postpartum period and thus makes up the lochia?
   A. decidua capsularis
   B. decidua vera
   C. decidua basalis
   D. none of the above   (4:108, 359−60)

10. How long does it take for the inner surface of the uterus, except for the placental site, to be covered with new epithelium?
   A. about 10 days
   B. about 3 weeks
   C. about 4 weeks
   D. about 6 weeks   (2:201)

11. Following complete involution the uterus should weigh about
   A. 12 oz
   B. 8 oz
   C. 6 oz
   D. 2 oz   (8:467)

12. The regrowth of the endometrial surface is analogous to what phase of the menstrual cycle?
   A. follicular
   B. luteal
   C. menstrual
   D. none of the above   (6:339)

13. The discomfort of after pains may be relieved by
   A. asking the woman to gently massage her abdomen
   B. asking the woman to lie on her side
   C. telling the woman that the after pains are not that severe
   D. suggesting that the woman lie on her abdomen   (3:602)

14. Which process prohibits the formation of scar tissue at the placental site?
   A. autolysis
   B. exfoliation
   C. self-digestion
   D. none of the above   (2:201)

15. Immediately after delivery, the cervix will admit
   A. one finger
   B. fingertip
   C. the hand
   D. two fingers   (8:468)

16. The cervix
   A. returns to a prepregnant state
   B. closes completely by the end of six weeks
   C. heals by process of the manufacture of new cells
   D. heals by process of involution   (4:360)

17. What is the name of the lochia that contains particles of decidua and cellular debris?
   A. rubra
   B. serosa
   C. alba
   D. none of the above   (4:360)

18. The lochia that contains a high amount of leukocytes is the
   A. rubra
   B. serosa
   C. alba
   D. none of the above   (3:599)

19. Which of the following might indicate subinvolution of the uterus?
   A. early onset of lochia serosa
   B. uterus decreasing in size
   C. lochia rubra extending into fifth day
   D. lochia alba extending into fourth week
                                     (3:599)

20. Lochia continues for approximately
   A. one week
   B. two weeks

C. three weeks
D. four weeks (7:131)

21. The ragged edges that replace the hymenal ring and persist after delivery are called

A. paramesonephric strands
C. carunculae myritiformes
C. lithokelyphos
D. rugae (8:469)

22. What is the name of the muscle that may become separated during pregnancy as a result of inadequate rest, exercise, and posture?

A. oblique muscle
B. rectus muscle
C. transverse muscle
D. ischiocavernosus muscle (3:597—8)

23. The breast milk usually "comes in" on the

A. first to second day
B. third to fourth day
C. fourth to fifth day
D. at delivery (4:361)

24. The discomfort associated with the filling of the breasts with milk is due primarily to increased tension in the area as a result of

A. increasing amounts of milk
B. increased circulation of blood and lymph in the mammary gland
C. above average fluid intake
D. process of involution (4:361)

25. The intense hunger following delivery is primarily due to

A. released pressure on the abdominal cavity
B. prolonged starvation period as a result of the laboring process
C. expended energies during labor
D. vomiting that occurs during labor (5:154)

26. Which of the following findings would be considered abnormal in the urine of a woman during the first 24 hours post partum?

A. lactose
B. 7 g nitrogen
C. acetone
D. none of the above (5:141)

27. Which of the following is considered to be a normal leukocyte count after the first postpartal week?

A. 30,000
B. 15,000
C. 10,000
D. 5,000 (5:154)

28. Which of the following hormones antepartally is primarily responsible for preparing the alveoli for its role in lactation?

A. estrogen
B. progesterone
C. somatomammotropin
D. lactogen (3:598)

29. A febrile condition is said to exist when a postpartum patient's temperature becomes elevated above

A. 100.4°F in any two consecutive 24-hour periods excluding the first 24 hours
B. 100.4°F in any two consecutive 24-hour periods starting at time of delivery
C. 99°F in any 24-hour period following delivery
D. 99°F in any two consecutive 24-hour periods excluding the first 24 hours (6:370)

30. The most common cause of a temperature rise during the first 20 hours following delivery is

A. chills
B. starvation
C. dehydration
D. strep infection (3:601)

31. If the nurse finds the fundus of the uterus enlarged, she should

A. check the consistency of the fundus after a 15-minute interval
B. massage the fundus vigorously with the open hand until it is below the umbilicus
C. keep the hand on the fundus until it becomes firm
D. massage the fundus firmly with the open hand while supporting uterus with the other hand (4:370—1)

32. Involution of the uterus is caused by

A. fatty degeneration of myometrial cells
B. necrosis of the hypertrophied muscle cells that are castoffs in the lochia
C. a breakdown of the protein material within the uterine wall, its absorption and fluid excretion in the urine
D. degeneration of the placental site and a decrease in the placental number of cells joined during pregnancy (8:468)

33. Although lochia varies in amount, it is generally most profuse in
   A. primiparas
   B. multiparas
   C. elderly primiparas
   D. cesarean section mothers   (4:360)

34. After pains during the postpartum period are the result of
   A. reflex contraction of the myometrium
   B. contraction and relaxation of the uterine muscle
   C. application of tension to uterine ligaments
   D. distention of the uterine vessels   (4:362)

35. As a rule, the fundus of the uterus on the third postpartum day should be palpated at which of the following levels?
   A. three or four fingers below the umbilicus
   B. one finger below the umbilicus
   C. at the level of the umbilicus
   D. at the symphysis pubis   (8:478)

36. Lochia rubra is
   A. colorless and transparent
   B. red
   C. pink, serous, or watery
   D. serous, milky, or ivory-colored   (8:468)

37. Subinvolution may be defined as the
   A. return of the uterus to a position not palpable in the abdomen
   B. retardation of the uterus to return to its original proportions
   C. failure of the uterus to return to its prepregnant state following oxytocin therapy
   D. inward folding of the fundus of the uterus to meet the cervical orifice   (8:531)

38. Postpartal "blues" are usually attributed to
   A. changes in hormonal levels
   B. ego regression
   C. fatigue, discomfort, and exhaustion
   D. all of the above   (4:370)

39. When caring for the perineum, whether the nurse or the patient carries out the procedure, it is most important to remember
   A. it is a sterile procedure
   B. all strokes go from front to back
   C. cleaning is carried out as for a catheterization
   D. to apply a sterile perineal pad   (4:376—7)

40. Sugar in the urine of the woman during the early postpartum period
   A. is usually indicative of diabetes mellitus
   B. may be the result of gestational diabetes
   C. is lactose, which is produced by the mammary glands
   D. none of the above   (3:602)

41. After pains may be the result of
   A. drugs given to stimulate the uterus to contract
   B. infant's sucking at the breast
   C. particles of cotyledons and blood clots that remain in the uterus
   D. all of the above   (6:341—2)

42. Which of the following measures is *not* helpful in relieving the discomfort associated with breast engorgement?
   A. wearing a snug binder
   B. use of a breast pump
   C. application of ice bag
   D. none of the above   (8:486)

43. Perineal sutures are absorbed in about
   A. three days
   B. five days
   C. one week to ten days
   D. two weeks   (6:341)

44. Urinary frequency during the first few days postpartum is likely to be indicative of
   A. postpartum cystitis
   B. a nervous response
   C. the body's effort to return its water metabolism to normal
   D. a temporary imbalance by the antidiuretic hormones   (4:363)

45. Which of the following factors predispose a woman to "diastasis of the rectus muscles"?
   1. premature infant
   2. multiple gestation
   3. grand multiparity
   4. a very large infant
   5. child with club feet

   A. 1, 2, 3
   B. 1, 3, 5
   C. 2, 3, 4
   D. all of the above   (6:342)

46. Recommended treatment for "diastasis of the recti muscles" is
    1. surgery
    2. prolonged bedrest
    3. good body mechanics
    4. ample rest
    5. exercises
    A. 1, 2, 3
    B. 2, 3, 4
    C. 3, 4, 5
    D. none of the above (6:342)

47. Following delivery, the empty uterus weighs approximately
    A. ½ lb
    B. 1 lb
    C. 1½ lb
    D. 2 lb (6:340)

48. On the day following delivery, the fundus is usually palpated
    A. one finger breadth above the umbilicus
    B. at the level of the umbilicus
    C. one finger breadth below the umbilicus
    D. two finger breadths below the umbilicus (8:478)

49. A slower pulse rate during the early puerperium
    A. is indicative of shock
    B. is a sign that an infection is present
    C. means that the woman is dehydrated
    D. is a transient phenomenon (4:362)

50. The woman who is *not* breast feeding can expect to have a return of her menstrual flow within what time period following delivery of her child?
    A. two weeks
    B. four weeks
    C. six weeks
    D. eight weeks (4:363)

51. During the "taking-in" phase, the woman's primary concerns are with
    A. herself
    B. her husband and other children
    C. her baby
    D. her own mother (3:586)

52. The taking in phase is one in which the mother
    A. wants to assume full responsibility for her child
    B. is quite talkative

C. wants to assume full responsibility for her own care
D. wants to be left alone (3:586)

53. The mother, in reviewing her labor and delivery experience, is
    A. showing neurotic tendencies
    B. seeking attention
    C. attempting to integrate it with reality
    D. seeking sympathy (4:363)

54. The "taking-hold" phase usually occurs
    A. about the second day, when the mother is able to get up to the bathroom and take care of herself
    B. about the first day, after the mother has a short rest and is ready to feed her baby for the first time
    C. about the third day, when the mother has moved from the passive individual to the one who is in command of the situation
    D. about the fifth day, when the mother is discharged home with her new child (4:367—8)

55. During the mother's early attempts to feed her baby, the nurse can be of greatest assistance by
    A. allowing the mother to feed the baby by herself, as the presence of an "expert" might increase the mother's self-consciousness
    B. telling the mother that the baby will be fed in the nursery if she (mother) experiences difficulty
    C. feeding the baby in front of the mother so that she (mother) can learn by watching
    D. encouraging the mother to feed the baby herself and then reinforcing correct behavior (4:369—70)

56. The taking-hold phase lasts
    A. 5 days
    B. 10 days
    C. 15 days
    D. 20 days (3:587)

57. The nurse can *best* meet the needs of the woman during the early postpartum period by
    A. remaining with her for long periods of time and providing the help for which she asks
    B. explaining to the woman that she is now basically on her own

C. leaving her alone but responding to the call for help immediately

D. telling the woman she is available and if anything is needed to ring the bell (8:474)

58. On the seventh postpartum day, the uterus should weigh about

A. 28 oz
B. 20 oz
C. 16 oz
D. 8 oz (4:360)

59. During the early postpartal days, the mother may experience problems associated with constipation because of

A. fluid imbalance
B. relaxed intestinal tone
C. relaxed abdominal muscles
D. all of the above (3:602)

60. Which drug is fairly commonly used to prevent lactation?

A. deladomane
B. diethylstilbestrol
C. Ergotrate
D. none of the above (8:415)

61. Following discharge from the hospital, women are usually requested to return to the doctor for an examination

A. two weeks postpartum
B. three weeks after discharge
C. four weeks after discharge
D. six weeks postpartum (8:450)

62. The new mother's first bath should be

A. done by the mother because she is used to providing care for herself
B. done by the mother because she needs to regain her independence as quickly as possible
C. done by the nurse because the mother is not physically and emotionally able to do it herself
D. done by the nurse because the mother needs to conserve energy (4:373)

63. An inability to void following delivery may be the result of

A. impaired tone of the bladder
B. decreased sensitiveness of the bladder
C. weak abdominal wall
D. all of the above (8:482)

64. During early puerperium, the diet should contain about how many calories per day?

A. 2,400 to 2,600
B. 2,600 to 2,800
C. 2,200 to 2,400
D. 2,000 to 2,200 (5:161)

65. The woman who has had varicosities of the veins should

A. be on complete bed rest for several days
B. apply Ace bandages to her legs before arising
C. sit on the side of the bed with her feet dangling several times each day
D. have a foot board on her bed (5:161)

66. Which of the following exercises is usually taught first to the postpartum mother?

A. lying on the side
B. lying on the abdomen
C. knee-chest position
D. none of the above (5:162)

67. The woman who is breast feeding should have a daily fluid intake of between

A. 1,500 to 2,000 mL
B. 2,000 to 2,500 mL
C. 2,500 to 3,000 mL
D. 3,000 to 3,500 mL (2:210)

68. Striae gravidarum eventually

A. heal
B. break open
C. become silvery white
D. go away (3:597)

69. Which of the following may be helpful in stimulating the bladder to empty?

A. having the mother breathe into a paper bag
B. having the mother blow bubbles through a straw into a glass of water
C. having the mother stand on the floor in her bare feet
D. having the mother sit on the bed pan for a long period of time (3:603)

70. Which of the following conditions is considered to be normal during the postpartum period?

A. nose bleeds
B. night sweats
C. shortness of breath
D. none of the above (3:604)

71. Ice packs are applied to the perineum during the first day postpartum to

    A. prevent or decrease edema of the episiotomy
    B. lessen the bleeding from the episiotomy
    C. prevent contact between the episiotomy and the perineal pad
    D. provide a contrairritant to the painful area   (3:604)

72. The milk-ejection reflex is the same as the

    A. expulsion mechanism
    B. letdown reflex
    C. draught reflex
    D. all of the above   (4:380)

73. Under stress, the letdown reflex can be inhibited. This occurs because of the action of

    A. estrogen
    B. oxytocin
    C. epinephrine
    D. none of the above   (6:414)

74. Which of the following may assist in restoring a declining milk flow?

    A. syntocinon
    B. estrogen
    C. thyroid
    D. none of the above   (6:414)

75. Which of the following best explains the letdown reflex?

    A. removal of milk from the breast by compression or suction
    B. release of luteotropic hormone, causing acini cells to produce milk
    C. release of oxytocin, causing cells around alveoli to force milk from alveoli and small ducts to larger ducts opening through the nipple
    D. release of luteotropic hormone, causing contraction of alveoli cells, which in turn cause milk to be propelled from small to larger ducts opening through the nipple   (4:380)

76. The pituitary hormone that acts to stimulate lactation in the face of diminishing circulation of estrogen and progesterone is

    A. FSH
    B. LH
    C. ADH
    D. LTH   (4:380)

77. Approximately how much calcium does the lactating mother lose daily?

    A. 25 mg
    B. 50 mg
    C. 75 mg
    D. none of the above   (6:348)

78. The recommended daily caloric intake for the lactating mother is between

    A. 1,800 and 2,000 calories
    B. 2,000 and 2,200 calories
    C. 2,400 and 2,600 calories
    D. 2,800 and 3,000 calories   (6:348)

79. Lactogenesis is stimulated by an increase of which of the following hormones?

    A. estrogen
    B. progesterone
    C. luteotropin
    D. all of the above   (6:345)

80. The nurse who works in a rooming-in unit must have additional knowledge of

    A. prenatal nursing
    B. postpartum nursing
    C. child care
    D. newborn care   (7:128–9)

81. The woman who is breast feeding *should* wear a good supporting brassiere

    A. to prevent discomfort during engorgement
    B. to maintain a good body image
    C. to prevent undue stretching of the breast tissue
    D. if she feels like it   (7:131)

82. The new mother should understand that propping of the baby's bottle

    A. is all right as long as the bottle is placed in an appropriate holder
    B. can realistically save her time
    C. provides insufficient cuddling for emotional support of the infant
    D. none of the above   (7:132)

83. During the first attempt to breast feed the newborn infant is it *most* important for the nurse to

    A. remember that the infant should nurse for about five minutes on each breast
    B. make sure that the mother understands that this is primarily a learning time for both herself and her newborn

C. make every attempt to keep the child awake during the entire feeding period
D. encourage the mother to give the child glucose water following breast feeding
(7:134)

84. The letting-go phase is best described by which of the following statements? The mother
A. recognizes that she has gone through labor and delivery, and has a new child
B. accepts the baby as an individual with its own personality, and establishes new norms for herself, the baby, and her family
C. has regained control over her own body functioning and is ready to take control of her child's body functioning
D. begins to feel confident in feeding her infant and is ready to let her husband learn how to feed the infant (3:556—7)

85. Who uses the term "maternal time-lag" in speaking of initial maternal behavior?
A. Miles Newton
B. Joseph Rheingold
C. Gerald Caplan
D. Ernestine Wiedenbach (3:592)

86. The term "maternal time-lag" refers to the
A. mother's waiting period during the period of pregnancy
B. span of time required for a new mother to feel that the baby really belongs to her
C. time period between a mother's desire to become pregnant and actual conception
D. mother's waiting period following delivery until her first sight of her newborn infant (3:592)

87. Who originally described the phases of "taking in," "taking hold," and "letting go" in relationship to the postpartum period?
A. Gerald Caplan
B. Sylvia Bruce
C. Reva Rubin
D. none of the above (3:586)

88. In assisting the new mother to care for her new infant, the nurse would do well to keep which of the following factors in mind?
A. the new mother should learn the basic principles involved in the care of her infant
B. the new mother should come up to the expectations that the nurse has for her regarding infant care
C. the new mother should be able to perform satisfactorily in the basic skills involved in infant care
D. the new mother should attain a feeling of comfort with her new infant (3:595)

89. Breast feeding
A. is never a satisfactory method of birth control
B. has no effect on ovulation
C. can suppress ovulation for about 75 days
D. none of the above (3:607)

90. Which of the following instructions should be given to a mother regarding breast care?
A. wash your nipples with warm water prior to each feeding
B. wash your nipples with mild soap and water prior to each feeding
C. wash your nipples with a mild antiseptic prior to each feeding
D. wash your nipples once a day with warm water (3:608)

91. During the early breast feeding routines, if the mother asks what position she should take, the nurst can best respond by advising her to
A. lie on her side with the head of the bed slightly elevated
B. sit up in the bed with the head of the bed elevated
C. sit up in a chair with pillows supporting her back
D. none of the above (8:626)

92. What percentage of babies born in the United States are breast fed?
A. 5 to 10%
B. 10 to 25%
C. 15 to 20%
D. 25 to 50% (3:606)

93. Which of the following organizations probably provides the greatest amount of help to breast feeding mothers?
A. Maternity Center Association
B. La Leche League
C. Childbirth Education Association
D. Psychoprophylatic Association (3:606)

94. The primary purpose of alternate massage is to
   A. dry the breast
   B. empty the breasts as completely as possible
   C. prevent primary engorgement
   D. supply breast milk for an infant who can not nurse at the breast   (3:612)

95. The best time to wean the infant from the breast is
   A. at about 6 weeks
   B. at about 12 weeks
   C. at about 6 months
   D. primarily up to the mother   (3:618)

96. All other factors being equal, which of the following factors would be most likely to produce a woman's emotional lag in response to her baby?
   A. a normal spontaneous delivery
   B. cesarean section under spinal anesthesia
   C. Lamaze method delivery
   D. delivery under deep anesthesia   (6:360)

97. The woman who experiences problems during labor and delivery will probably
   A. want to begin caring for her child at once
   B. want to give her child up for adoption
   C. want to rest and recover without the child for about the first day
   D. want the child to be fed in the nursery during her hospital stay   (6:360)

98. The nurse can best help the mother who is experiencing a maternal time-lag by
   A. meeting mother's needs and demonstrating warmth toward the infant while in the presence of the mother
   B. providing major care for the infant during the entire hospital stay
   C. insisting that the mother start to provide care for her infant immediately
   D. leaving the mother alone with her infant so that the mother can work out her own role with the infant   (3:592)

99. Mothers who do not show instant love toward their infant
   A. are not normal and should not be allowed to provide care to their child without supervision
   B. may feel guilt and should be helped to see that this is normal

C. do not have the capacity to become a mother and should give up the child
   D. are immature and should be referred for further help   (3:591−2)

100. Which of the following maternal behavior, observed during pregnancy, usually results in a shortened maternal time-lag during the puerperium?
   A. nausea and vomiting
   B. talking to unborn child
   C. maternal conflicts
   D. none of the above   (3:593)

101. The mother who develops a strong attachment to her unborn child during pregnancy
   A. may reject the child at birth
   B. experiences problems during the taking-in phase
   C. experiences problems during the taking-hold phase
   D. experiences problems during the letting-go phase   (3:593)

102. Which of the following actions would the nurse probably see when the mother receives her infant for the first time?
   A. she eagerly reaches for the child, undresses and examines it completely
   B. her arms and hands are used passively to receive the child, she then traces his profile with her fingertips
   C. her arms and hands are used passively to receive the child, she then holds the child to her own body
   D. she eagerly reaches for the child, then holds the child close to her own body   (6:360−1)

103. The mother who has delivered by cesarean section needs to know that in most cases she will be unable to breast feed immediately after delivery because of
   A. the prolonged delay in the onset of lactation
   B. the discomfort caused by the incision
   C. the infant's response to the delivery with the resulting weak sucking reflex
   D. none of the above   (6:367)

104. Which of the following are considered to be appropriate for the postpartum mother during her first week at home?
   1. may go up and down stairs
   2. rest most of the day to avoid fatigue
   3. continue with exercises practiced in hospital

4. care for herself and baby only
5. should have scanty lochia

A. 1, 2, 3, 4
B. 2, 3, 4
C. 2, 3, 4, 5
D. all of the above   (6:349)

105. After delivery, how long should the woman abstain from coitus?

A. one week
B. two weeks
C. four weeks
D. six weeks   (6:349)

106. In considering the mother-infant relationship, the nurse should be aware that

1. maternal touch is an index of how the mother feels about herself and her relation to the baby
2. most mothers need reassurance regardless of parity and type of delivery
3. most mothers express dependency needs in the early postpartal period
4. there may be a need on the part of the mother to express feelings of loss about the birth of the child

A. 1, 2
B. 1, 2, 3
C. 3
D. all of the above   (3:591—5)

107. Puerperal infection may be defined as

A. a postpartum wound infection of the birth canal
B. an infection of the uterine cavity
C. a postpartum infection of the birth canal, occurring secondarily to another infection in the baby
D. any infection occurring within six weeks of delivery   (4:515)

108. Puerperal infections are most commonly caused by

A. colon bacillus
B. staphylococcus
C. streptococcus
D. Welch bacillus   (4:515)

109. The two main predisposing causes of puerperal infection are

A. hemorrhage and dehydration
B. chills and hemorrhage
C. hemorrhage and trauma
D. trauma and dehydration   (4:515)

110. Puerperal fever is most likely to be contracted by the woman because of

A. prolonged ruptured membranes
B. poor hygiene on the woman's part
C. poor technique on the part of medical and nursing staff
D. unsterile equipment in labor and delivery room and on postpartum unit   (4:515—16)

111. Endometritis during the postpartum period may be considered a

A. local lesion process
B. extension of the original lesion process
C. an infection of unknown cause
D. none of the above   (4:517)

112. Endometritis usually occurs during what time period following the delivery?

A. 6 to 12 hours
B. 12 to 24 hours
C. 24 to 48 hours
D. 48 to 72 hours   (4:517)

113. Which of the following symptoms might suggest that a woman has endometritis?

A. large boggy uterus; red lochia, moderate amount
B. large tender uterus; brown lochia, small amount
C. small uterus; red lochia, large amount
D. small uterus; pink lochia, small amount   (4:517)

114. Endometritis that remains localized usually lasts about

A. two to three days
B. five days to a week
C. one week to ten days
D. about two weeks   (4:517)

115. The most common localized infection following delivery is found in the

A. uterus
B. perineum
C. loose connective tissue
D. vascular endothelium   (4:517)

116. The preferred drug in endometritis is

A. Darvon
B. penicillin
C. ergonovine
D. Pitocin   (4:517—8)

117. Thrombophlebitis is
   A. a localized infection of the peritoneum
   B. an infection of the vascular endothelium
   C. an infection of the vascular endothelium with clot formation attached to the vessel wall
   D. a generalized infection of the perineum
   (4:518)

118. Which of the following statements best describes pelvic thrombophlebitis?
   A. pain and swelling in the affected leg on about the tenth day postpartum
   B. chills, general malaise, head- and backaches
   C. repeated chills, dramatic swings in temperature
   D. dorsiflexion of foot and pressure over deep veins causes pain in the calf of the leg
   (4:519)

119. Peritonitis may result when
   A. the infection travels from the endometrium to the peritoneum via the lymphatic vessels
   B. there is an extension of thrombophlebitis or parametritis
   C. both A and B
   D. neither A nor B
   (4:519)

120. The causative agent in puerperal fever was probably first seen by
   A. Mayrhofer in 1863
   B. Pasteur in 1879
   C. Holmes in 1843
   D. Semmelweiss in 1861
   (4:662)

121. Oliver Wendell Holmes is to the nature of puerperal fever as Semmelweiss is to
   A. the cause of child-bed fever
   B. obstetrical forceps
   C. the transmission of puerperal fever
   D. internal podalic version
   (4:661)

122. Who is responsible for the introduction of sterile rubber gloves and thus the reduction of puerperal infection?
   A. Louis Pasteur
   B. Oliver Wendell Holmes
   C. Dr. Halsted
   D. none of the above
   (8:523)

123. Who wrote *The Etiology, Conception and Prophylaxis of Child-Bed Fever*?
   A. Holmes
   B. Semmelweiss
   C. Pasteur
   D. Halsted
   (8:523)

124. Which of the following is considered to be a preventive measure against puerperal infection?
   A. hand washing by all personnel
   B. deliveries under sterile technique
   C. elimination of staff with bacterial respiratory infections
   D. all of the above
   (8:526)

125. Which of the following is considered to be a complication of pelvic thrombophlebitis?
   A. lung abscess
   B. pleurisy
   C. pneumonia
   D. all of the above
   (3:758)

126. Thrombophlebitis is often referred to as
   A. "milk leg"
   B. phlegmasia alba aldens
   C. both A and B
   D. neither A nor B
   (3:759)

127. Which drug is most frequently used in superficial femoral thrombophlebitis?
   A. heparin
   B. penicillin
   C. streptomycin
   D. none of the above
   (3:759)

128. The causative organism in pelvic thrombophlebitis is most often
   A. *Staphylococcus aureus*
   B. anaerobic streptococcus
   C. hemolytic streptococcus
   D. colon bacillus
   (3:758)

129. The symptoms of femoral thrombophlebitis usually occur about
   A. twelve hours after delivery
   B. two days postpartum
   C. the tenth day postpartum
   D. none of the above
   (4:518)

130. Which of the following veins are involved in pelvic thrombophlebitis?
   1. uterine
   2. hypogastric
   3. saphenous
   4. popliteal
   5. ovarian

   A. 1, 2, 3
   B. 1, 2, 5
   C. 2, 3, 4
   D. none of the above
   (6:372)

131. Which of the following symptoms are usually associated with peritonitis?
   A. malaise followed by stiffness and pain in affected area
   B. fever, redness, and edema of the area
   C. high fever, rapid pulse, constant abdominal pain
   D. onset—second week—repeated chills, swings in temperature   (4:519)

132. The drug of choice in treating the hemolytic streptococcus is
   A. penicillin
   B. sulfadiazine
   C. Gantrisin
   D. erythromycin   (4:520)

133. During the immediate postpartum period, the woman with diabetes will need
   A. more insulin than during the pregnancy
   B. less insulin than was needed during pregnancy
   C. about the same amount of insulin that was needed during pregnancy
   D. none of the above   (3:760)

134. Which of the following conditions will increase the possibility of mastitis?
   A. fissured nipples
   B. bruising of breast tissue
   C. stasis of milk in a milk duct
   D. all of the above   (8:529)

135. Mastitis in the postpartum period usually occurs
   A. during the first three to five days postpartum
   B. during first week of postpartum period
   C. between first and fourth week of the puerperium
   D. during the sixth week following birth of the infant   (8:529)

136. Which of the following would be fairly likely to occur prior to the onset of mastitis?
   A. gradual drying of the breast milk
   B. complete emptying of both breasts
   C. marked engorgement of the breasts
   D. nonlactating breasts   (4:523)

137. Mastitis can be prevented by
   A. good prenatal care of the breasts
   B. good postpartum care of the breasts
   C. observation and treatment of sores and cracks of nipples
   D. all of the above   (4:523)

138. The source of infection of epidemic puerperal breast abscess is
   A. cracked nipples
   B. contaminated hands
   C. inverted nipples
   D. the infant   (4:524)

139. Cystitis during the puerperium is due to
   A. bladder trauma
   B. stagnant residual urine
   C. bacteria that have entered the bladder
   D. all of the above   (8:531)

140. Cystitis in the postpartum woman can be suspected if the woman has
   A. suprapubic or perineal discomfort, frequent and painful urination
   B. pain in the flank, frequency of urination
   C. severe lower backache and urinary retention
   D. none of the above   (8:531)

141. The woman with cardiac disease should be observed for which of the following signs during the first two days postpartum?
   A. edema
   B. changes in apical pulse
   C. rate of respirations
   D. all of the above   (3:756)

142. When bleeding occurs immediately after the delivery of the placenta, which of the following causes should be considered first?
   A. uterine atony
   B. uterine lacerations
   C. rupture of the uterus
   D. retained membranes   (8:519)

143. Which of the following measures should be employed by the doctor if abdominal massage and oxytocins are not effective in controlling bleeding caused by uterine atony?
   A. hysterectomy
   B. internal bimanual compression
   C. external bimanual compression
   D. pack the uterus with gauze   (8:520)

144. Which of the following IV solutions would be given to a woman whenever it appears that blood loss will be above usual in order to maintain an adequate blood volume until blood can be obtained?
   A. dextrose 5% in water
   B. dextrose 5% in Ringer's lactate

C. dextrose 5% in saline
D. none of the above   (8:521)

145. An untreated gonorrheal infection in the postpartum woman can produce

A. sterility
B. severe headaches
C. very high fever
D. all of the above   (8:527)

146. Which of the following statements best describes the symptoms associated with a vulvar hematoma?

A. pain and sensation of heat in the area, and burning on urination
B. severe pain in the perineal area, feeling of pressure on the rectum and bladder
C. gradually rising fundus during the first hours following delivery with small amount of lochia rubra
D. edema of the perineal area following a second laceration and repair   (6:373)

147. Vulvar hematomas are likely to occur

A. following a rapid spontaneous delivery
B. following prolonged pressure during labor and delivery
C. in patients who have large varicosities in the pelvic area
D. all of the above   (6:373)

148. Passive immunization of hemolytic disease caused by Rh incompatibility can be obtained through the use of

A. vaccinia virus
B. RhoGAM
C. packed red blood cells
D. none of the above   (8:732)

149. Which of the following doctors was responsible for the discovery of RhoGAM?

A. Freda
B. Gorman
C. Pollack
D. all of the above   (6:375)

150. When was RhoGAM offered to the general public?

A. 1964
B. 1966
C. 1968
D. 1970   (6:375)

151. RhoGAM is usually given

A. on first prenatal visit
B. on thirty-fourth week of pregnancy

C. at onset of labor
D. within 72 hours after delivery   (8:732)

152. What is the standard dose of RhoGAM?

A. 50 to 75 μg IM
B. 150 to 200 μg IU
C. 200 to 300 μg IM
D. 400 to 500 μg IV   (6:376)

153. Which of the following increase the possibility of immunization of Rh negative mothers by Rh positive fetal blood?

A. oxytocin-induced labor
B. abortion
C. hydatidiform mole
D. all of the above   (6:375)

154. The woman who has complications during the early puerperium will probably have a

A. shortened taking-hold phase
B. prolonged taking-in phase
C. delayed letting-go phase
D. precipitate letting-go phase   (3:746)

155. Subinvolution is usually caused by

A. retained placental fragments
B. lack of muscle tone
C. endometritis
D. all of the above   (4:521)

156. Which of the following descriptions best describes the symptoms observed in subinvolution?

A. small uterus, lochia alba for two weeks
B. large, tender uterus, small amount foul lochia, brownish color
C. large uterus, lochia profuse and prolonged
D. small uterus, lochia rubra on third day
              (4:521)

157. Late postpartal hemorrhage is most commonly caused by

A. clots within the uterus
B. episiotomy dehiscence
C. retained placental fragments
D. uterine muscle atrophy   (8:521)

158. The woman should have her blood pressure checked daily because of

A. possible shock resulting from loss of blood
B. possible elevation due to oxytocic drugs she may be receiving
C. possible toxemia which can occur during the postpartum period
D. none of the above   (2:208)

159. Which of the following are used to provide temporary relief of painful sutures in the perineal area?

A. dermoplast
B. americaine
C. tucks
D. all of the above (2:211)

160. The highest number of postpartum hemorrhages occur

A. during the first 12 hours
B. from 12 to 24 hours after delivery
C. from the second to third postpartum day
D. none of the above (2:231)

161. The drug of choice in subinvolution is

A. sparteine sulfate
B. Methergine
C. Pitocin
D. Syntocinon (4:521)

162. The incidence of vulvar or vaginal hematomas is about once in every

A. 100 to 500 cases
B. 500 to 1,000 cases
C. 750 to 1,500 cases
D. 1,000 to 1,750 cases (4:521)

163. A complete absence of mammary secretion is known as

A. hypogalactia
B. agalactia
C. galactorrhea
D. polygalactia (4:522)

164. The ability to produce breast milk is dependent upon

A. the individual's general health
B. physical appearance of the breasts
C. degree of development of the glandular portions of the breasts
D. all of the above (4:522)

165. Mastitis is most frequently the result of which organisms?

A. staphylococcus
B. streptococcus
C. colon bacillus
D. Welch bacillus (8:529)

166. The woman who is awake during the delivery process is usually aware of any problems associated with her new infant. She senses this through

A. the staff's change in verbal communication with her

B. the staff's attempts to use their bodies to block her view of the baby
C. the staff's rigid posture
D. all of the above (4:583)

167. Parents frequently do not ask for particular details regarding their newborn infant because

A. they are afraid to ask, fearing that they will find out that there is something really wrong with the child
B. they would rather wait until the professional person has time to sit down and discuss it with them
D. they are too excited to care about any problems which might exist
D. they are well prepared for parenthood and already know what to expect (7:146)

168. Professionals do not always tell parents about the abnormalities present in the newborn child because

A. they are afraid of the reactions the parents might have
B. they feel that the parents might worry too much
C. they feel that the problems should be handled as they arise
D. all of the above (7:146)

169. Following the birth of a premature infant, the parents are probably *most* concerned about

A. the increased hospital and medical costs that will be involved
B. the problems mentioned in giving care to the infant
C. the viability and continued existence of the infant
D. none of the above (3:751)

170. The parents' initial response to the notification that their newborn infant has died will be one of

A. disbelief and shock
B. feelings of pain and anguish
C. acceptance of the death
D. none of the above (3:674−6)

171. If the mother does not see her less-than-perfect child in the delivery room

A. she will deny that the child is hers when she does see it
B. she will forget that the child has any deviations from normal

C. she will have increased fantasies about the child
D. none of the above   (3:751−2)

Directions: Each group of numbered words or phrases is followed by a list of lettered statements. MATCH the lettered statement with the numbered word or phrase most closely associated with it.

Questions 172 through 175
172. ragged edges of tissue that replace the hymenal ring after childbirth
173. separation of the recti muscles
174. process by which involution takes place
175. normal pulse rate during the early puerperium

A. bradycardia
B. autolysis
C. carunculae myrtiformes
D. diastasis   (6:342; 8:468)

Questions 176 through 179
176. absence or failure of secretion of milk
177. causing the flow of milk
178. excessive flow of milk
179. maintenance of milk

A. galactorrhea
B. galactopoiesis
C. agalactia
D. galactagogue   (4:681,684; 6:345)

Questions 180 through 182
180. a localized infection of the lining membrane of the uterus
181. a localized infection of the inner muscular layer of the uterus
182. an infection involving the peritoneum and broad ligament
183. a generalized or local infection of the peritoneum

A. endomyometritis
B. parametritis
C. endometritis
D. peritonitis   (4:517−9; 6:371)

Directions: This part of the test consists of a situation followed by a series of questions and incomplete statements. Study the situation and select the BEST answer in each case.

Questions 184 through 197
Mrs. Jane Johnson, gravida 1, para 1, age 24, delivered a full-term living female infant approximately four hours ago. She had a median episiotomy and the infant weighed 7 lb, 2 oz at birth. You are the nurse caring for Mrs. Johnson.

184. Mrs. Johnson's fundus is three fingers above the umbilicus to the right side and boggy. You would *first*

A. have her turn to her side
B. vigorously massage the fundus for five minutes
C. have her void
D. realize there is no reason for concern since this a common reaction four hours after delivery   (4:373−4)

185. Mrs. Johnson turns to you and says, "I saw the baby in the recovery room. She sure has a pointed head." Which of the following statements would be the best response?

A. "Yes, that's because your pelvis was almost too small for the baby's head to pass through."
B. "That is molding. It is transitory and the head will be nice and round in several days."
C. "All babies are that way. They use their head to push their way out."
D. "Oh, if she had more hair you wouldn't notice that."   (2:246−7)

186. Mrs. Johnson asks how soon she may get up and shower. In discussing early ambulation with Mrs. Johnson, you should keep in mind the main *disadvantage* of early ambulation, which is

A. increasing chance of hemorrhage
B. increasing incidence of thrombophlebitis
C. slowing the rate of involution
D. increasing the chances of overexertion   (4:372−3)

187. The first two days post partum, Mrs. Johnson will most likely have which kind of vaginal discharge?

A. lochia serosa
B. lochia rubra
C. lochia sangre
D. lochia alba   (8:479)

188. When Mrs. Johnson asks you why she had to have an episiotomy, you would probably offer which of the following explanations?

A. with your first baby you always need an episiotomy because the opening hasn't been stretched before
B. an episiotomy is usually done because the baby's head is so big it won't come out any other way

C. an episiotomy is performed when the vaginal opening is already as large as it can be without tearing your muscles
D. it reduces the stress on your baby during the second stage and reduces the stress on your perineum and other organs (4:349)

You enter Mrs. Johnson's room on her first postpartum day. Which of the following observations would indicate that Mrs. Johnson is progressing normally?

189. Breasts
    1. soft
    2. engorged
    3. secreting colostrum
    4. secreting milk
    5. not secreting any fluid

    A. 2, 3
    B. 1, 5
    C. 2, 4
    D. 1, 3 (4:361)

190. Fundus
    1. soft
    2. firm
    3. at the level of the umbilicus
    4. midway between the umbilicus and symphysis pubis
    5. at the level of the symphysis pubis

    A. 1, 2
    B. 1, 5
    C. 2, 3
    D. 2, 5 (8:478)

191. Lochia
    1. blood mixed with small amount of mucus
    2. characteristic foul odor
    3. fleshy odor
    4. clear-colored, moderate amount
    5. dark brown with occasional red bleeding

    A. 1, 2
    B. 1
    C. 2, 3
    D. 3, 5 (8:468)

192. Perineum
    1. edematous
    2. painful to pressure
    3. intense pain in the area
    4. clear discharge
    5. hemorrhoids

    A. 1, 2, 4
    B. 2, 3, 4

C. 1, 2, 5
D. all of the above (8:481)

193. Temperature and pulse
    A. T 100° and P 92
    B. T 98° and P 60
    C. T 98° and P 82
    D. T 101° and P 96 (8:470)

194. Two days after delivery, Mrs. Johnson begins to feel uncomfortable, with heavy, tender breasts. She wears a well-fitting bra, but the engorgement is still very pronounced. This engorgement is mainly due to

    A. excessive production of milk
    B. inadequate intake-output balance
    C. increased circulation of blood and lymph in mammary tissue
    D. subinvolution (4:361)

195. Mrs. Johnson asks if breast feeding may be considered a reliable contraceptive measure as long as she does not have a menstrual period. Which of the following responses would be most appropriate?

    A. some mothers have found breast feeding to be a good way to space their children
    B. yes, breast feeding may be used as a contraceptive measure until the return of normal periods
    C. breast feeding should not be considered a reliable contraceptive measure
    D. breast feeding is ineffective as a contraceptive measure because the return of a normal period varies with each mother (3:607)

196. Mrs. Johnson's protein requirement will be greatest in the

    A. first trimester of pregnancy
    B. second trimester of pregnancy
    C. third trimester of pregnancy
    D. period following delivery (3:328)

197. Mrs. Johnson expresses concern about her ability to breast feed since her breasts are small. Your best response would be

    A. the size and shape of the breasts do not affect the milk secretion. It is the amount of glandular tissue in the breasts that is important
    B. yes, your breasts are small and this may make breast feeding difficult. Bottle feeding can be just as satisfying

C. it may be well for you to discuss this further with your doctor
D. it would be advantageous to try breast feeding despite the size of your breasts
(8:616)

Questions 198 through 213
Mrs. Sally Lancaster is a 29-year-old mother who was admitted to the postpartum unit approximately one hour ago. Her first child, a female, was born 3½ years ago by cesarean section. Although Mrs. Lancaster had been scheduled for an elective section at term for the present pregnancy, the onset of labor at the thirty-eighth week of gestation had resulted in the emergency section which was done six hours ago under spinal anesthesia. The baby, a boy, weighed 6 lb at birth and is in good condition. Mrs. Lancaster spent the last five hours in the recovery room. You are assigned to Mrs. Lancaster for her morning care.

198. Which of the following were probably included in Mrs. Lancaster's preoperative orders?
1. abdominal skin prep
2. Foley catheter insertion
3. morphine sulfate sc
4. atropine sc
5. enema

A. 1, 2, 3
B. 2, 4, 5
C. 1, 2, 4
D. all of the above (8:459—60)

199. Mrs. Lancaster had a low segment cesarean section. This means that
A. the uterus was removed following the section
B. after the abdomen was opened a transverse incision was made in the lower cervical segment of the uterus
C. one incision was made in the midline of the abdomen and another in the uterus longitudinally
D. the fallopian tubes were tied and cut following the section (6:331)

200. The mortality rate for an infant delivered by cesarean section in comparison to that of the child delivered by the vaginal route is
A. about the same
B. twice as high
C. half as great
D. four times as high (6:330)

201. Which of the following complications could arise in Mrs. Lancaster?
1. infection
2. hemorrhage
3. ileus
4. acute dilation of the stomach

A. 1, 2
B. 1, 2, 3
C. 3, 4
D. all of the above (8:460—1)

202. Which of the following would probably be included in the postoperative orders?
1. check vital signs every 5 minutes for 2 hours, then every 15 minutes until stable
2. connect Foley catheter to constant drainage
3. NPO for 24 hours and give IV 1,000 5% G/W first postpartum morning
4. encourage deep breathing, coughing, and turning in bed
5. Demerol 100 mg q.4h p.r.n. through first 24 hours

A. 1, 4, 5
B. 1, 2, 4
C. 3, 4, 5,
D. all of the above (4:456)

203. The orders for Mrs. Lancaster also indicate that she is to be kept flat for eight hours following the delivery. Why?
A. cerebrospinal fluid pressure is increased from the spinal and she will have a headache if she sits up
B. there may be leakage of spinal fluid from the dura
C. to allow the effects of the anesthesia to wear off
D. to allow her to get the sleep necessary for her restoration (4:372—3)

204. You enter Mrs. Lancaster's room. She is drowsy from her pain medication but opens her eyes as you approach her bed. She asks, "Is my baby all right?" Your best response would be to say
A. your baby is fine. You may see him at the next feeding period
B. try to get some rest now
C. I know that you would like to see your baby. The nurse will be bringing him out soon
D. your baby is fine. I will go and see if the nursery nurse can bring him in for you to see right now (6:330)

205. Mrs. Lancaster's abdominal bandage makes it impossible for you to palpate the uterus. However, you notice that there is no extensive bleeding. Which of the following signs would indicate that internal hemorrhage is occurring?

   A. decreased pulse, decreased respirations, drop in blood pressure
   B. increased pulse, increased respirations, drop in blood pressure
   C. drop in blood pressure
   D. increased pulse, decreased respirations
   (4:456)

206. Mrs. Lancaster may have a delayed recovery phase in

   A. the taking-in period
   B. the taking-hold period
   C. the letting-go period
   D. there is no reason why she should have a delayed recovery period (3:746)

207. Mrs. Lancaster is interested in breast feeding her infant and asks you when she will be able to start. Your best response would be to say

   A. it would be better for you and the child to wait until you are able to be up and around
   B. women who have had cesarean sections are usually too uncomfortable to breast feed their infants
   C. you may start whenever you feel that you are ready
   D. the child who is born by cesarean section is not usually fed for 16 hours. You may feed your infant after this amount of time has lapsed (5:278)

208. On the evening of the first postpartum day, Mrs. Lancaster is helped out of bed. In addition to the usual preparation for getting a patient out of bed, which of the following points should be *stressed*?

   1. early ambulation is necessary for your quick recovery
   2. there will be increased lochia with ambulation
   3. the incision will not break open with movement

   4. you will feel better if you get out of bed

   A. 1, 2
   B. 2, 3
   C. 1, 4
   D. 3, 4 (2:191−2)

209. Mrs. Lancaster will experience many of the same emotional and physical changes as the woman who delivers vaginally. Which of the following may *not* be experienced by Mrs. Lancaster?

   A. after pains
   B. breast engorgement
   C. satisfaction in the birth process
   D. taking-in phase (4:456)

210. Mrs. Lancaster may have particular problems with flatus on her third postpartum day. Which of the following may be helpful in relieving Mrs. Lancaster's discomfort?

   1. large amounts of iced drinks
   2. ambulation
   3. Harris flush
   4. rectal tube
   5. prostigmine

   A. 1, 2, 4, 5
   B. 1, 2, 3, 4
   C. 2, 3, 4, 5
   D. all of the above (2:192)

211. Mrs. Lancaster may have a lag in her maternal feelings because

   A. she had spinal anesthesia rather than general anesthesia
   B. she had an emergency section rather than an elective section
   C. both A and B
   D. neither A nor B (3:632)

212. Mrs. Lancaster will probably be discharged

   A. fifth to sixth postpartum day
   B. sixth to eighth postpartum day
   C. eighth to tenth postpartum day
   D. tenth to twelfth postpartum day (5:241)

213. Mrs. Lancaster will be asked to make an appointment with her doctor in

   A. one week
   B. two weeks
   C. three weeks
   D. six weeks (2:192)

Answers and Explanations: Postpartum Period

1. **B.** This period is usually spoken of as the six weeks following the birth of the infant.

2. **A.** Involution is a retrograde process of change by which the uterus becomes smaller.

3. **B.** Involution actually starts about two days after delivery.

4. **D.** The uterus weighs about 2 lb immediately after delivery.

5. **C.** The fundus then quickly rises to the level of the umbilicus.

6. **C.** A full bladder will raise the level of the umbilicus.

7. **C.** Finger breadths above or below the umbilicus is the usual method of measuring and recording.

8. **D.** After pains are most commonly experienced in multigravidas and in mothers who breast feed.

9. **D.** The decidua vera is that portion not in direct contact with the products of conception.

10. **A.** The uterus becomes lined with epithelium in about a week to ten days. Other authors indicate this may take three weeks.

11. **D.** By the end of the puerperium the uterus should return to its original position and size and weight, which is about 2 oz.

12. **A.** During the follicular phase, and under the influence of estrogen, the endometrium regenerates and grows. The follicular phase follows the menstrual phase.

13. **D.** This position may ease the discomfort of the after pains.

14. **B.** It is believed that a process of exfoliation brings about the disappearance of the obliterated arteries and organized thrombi and undermines the site of placental attachment.

15. **C.** The cervical canal gradually closes and will admit one finger at the end of a week.

16. **C.** The cervix heals by manufacture of new cells and never returns to its prepregnant state, that is, the external os remains open to a certain degree.

17. **A.** Lochia rubra is the first discharge and contains blood and substances from the placental site. This discharge lasts about three days.

18. **C.** The whitish-yellow color is due to the increased number of leukocytes.

19. **C.** An extended period of lochia rubra can indicate retained placental fragments.

20. **D.** Lochia continues for about a month, but there are variations depending on the individual woman.

21. **B.** Carunculae myrtiformes occur only during labor or the explusion of a large tumor, thus, they may offer proof that a woman has borne at least one child.

22. **B.** As a result the abdominal organs are not properly supported.

23. **B.** The breasts fill with milk on the third or fourth day following delivery.

24. **B.** This increased tension on the very sensitive surrounding tissues is sometimes termed primary engorgement.

25. **C.** Hunger needs are primarily due to the large amount of energy expended during the labor and delivery experience.

26. **D.** All of the findings mentioned are considered to be normal in the urine during the first 24 hours post partum.

27. **B.** This event is a defense against possible infections and also helps in body repair. Immediately following delivery the leukocyte count may be as high as 30,000.

28. **B.** Estrogen affects primarily the ducts. The exact role of somatomammotropin is unknown at this time.

29. **A.** Fever is the first cardinal symptom of puerperal infection to appear. Any temperature, however, between 99.5° and 100.4°F may be indicative of a beginning infection.

30. **C.** Women may have a low intake of fluids and may also perspire profusely during the laboring process.

31. **D.** Support of the lower portion of the uterus should be provided by applying slight pressure of the hand on the suprapubic area.

32. **C.** The secretion of these products increases the nitrogen content in the urine.

33. **B.** Also, ambulation for the first time increases the amount of lochia in all mothers.

34. **B.** After pains are more common in the multiparas than in the primiparas, because of the loss of muscle tone that occurs after a repeated pregnancy. Thus the muscle tends to contract and relax at intervals.

35. **A.** The height of the fundus descends gradually, and there is much individual difference in the descent. However, some authors indicate that it descends about one finger breadth per day.

36. **B.** During the first few days post partum, lochia rubra is bright red because of the large amount of blood in the discharge.

37. **C.** Subinvolution may be caused by retention of placental fragments as a part of the fetal membranes. It may also be caused by an endometritis.

38. **D.** Postpartal blues are usually a very temporary thing and may occur either in the hospital or following discharge.

39. **B.** Strokes that go from front to back will avoid the possibility of bringing the organisms that harbor around the rectal area forward to the birth canal.

40. **C.** Lactose is most frequently seen during the time of the establishment of the milk flow and also when the mother is weaning the child.

41. **D.** All of the factors mentioned may cause after pains in the woman.

42. **B.** The use of a breast pump to remove the milk simply stimulates the breasts to produce more milk.

43. **C.** The perineal sutures are absorbed in about a week to 10 days.

44. **C.** During pregnancy there is an increased tendency of the body to retain water, immediately post partum. The diuresis is the body's effort to return its water metabolism to normal.

45. **C.** Increased uterine pressure against the abdominal wall can cause a separation of the rectus muscles in the midline.

46. **C.** These measures will assist in restoring muscle tone.

47. **D.** Following delivery, the empty uterus weighs approximately 2 lb.

48. **B.** The fundus is often several finger breadths below the umbilicus immediately after delivery, and then rises to the level of the umbilicus where it may remain for a day or so.

49. **D.** A slower pulse rate during the early puerperium is a favorable sign, and usually by the end of 7 to 10 days the pulse returns to its normal rate.

50. **D.** The woman who is breast feeding *may* not have a menstrual period until lactation is discontinued, but this is not a certainty.

51. **A.** The new mother's concerns are primarily sleep and food.

52. **B.** The nurse can be of great help to the mother during this time. She can assist the mother by listening to and interpreting recent past events for both mother and father.

53. **C.** The new mother needs information about the labor and delivery experience so that she can form a total picture of what really happened during delivery. In this way she realizes that the delivery is really over and her baby has been born.

54. **C.** The mother now knows that she can regain control of her own body functioning and is now able to begin to assume responsibility for her new child.

55. **D.** By doing this, the nurse demonstrates that she has confidence in the mother's ability to cope with the new tasks.

56. **B.** The taking-hold phase is a time when the mother is taking hold of many things and striving to master new tasks. Teaching is thus an important aspect of nursing care.

57. **D.** The mother may not be able to express her needs directly or readily during this time and may benefit from an anticipation of these needs.

58. **C.** On the seventh postpartum day, the uterus should weight about 16 oz.

59. **D.** All of the factors mentioned can cause constipation in the postpartum woman.

60. **A.** Deladomane is a long-acting drug of estrogen-androgen combination.

61. **D.** The postpartum checkup is usually done six weeks after delivery. By this time the pelvic

organs should have returned to a normal condition.

62. **D.** This also allows the nurse to make additional physiologic observations about the woman that are helpful in further planning for her care.

63. **D.** All of the above-mentioned factors may lead to a woman's inability to void following delivery.

64. **B.** A diet high in proteins, vitamins, and minerals is essential for tissue repair and the mother's well-being.

65. **B.** Ace bandages prevent stasis and improve circulation. The mother should have early ambulation as this also aids in improving circulation.

66. **B.** This exercise helps strengthen the abdominal muscles and hastens involution. The mother may not be aware of this exercise unless she is told about it.

67. **C.** Increased fluid intake promotes milk production.

68. **C.** Striae gravidarum are "stretch" marks that appear on the abdomen and breasts.

69. **B.** A warm sitzbath, or pouring water slowly over the symphysis and labia also may help in stimulating the bladder to empty.

70. **B.** It is normal for the woman to have diaphoresis during the night. This is called "night sweats."

71. **A.** Edema of the perineum is the major cause of discomfort resulting from an episiotomy.

72. **D.** All of the terms mentioned refer to the second mechanism involved in lactation. The first mechanism is that of the secretion of milk.

73. **C.** Epinephrine is a vasoconstrictor and inhibits oxytocin from stimulating breast tissues.

74. **C.** Thyroid hormone may be given to increase a declining milk flow. Syntocinon is given to assist in the initial letdown of the milk. This drug causes the myoepithelium to contract and release the milk into the ducts.

75. **C.** The letdown reflex can be influenced by psychological factors and the emotions of the mother.

76. **B.** The lactogenic hormone is prolactin. This hormone is released from the anterior pituitary following separation and delivery of the placenta.

77. **D.** The lactating mother loses 150 to 300 mg of calcium in her milk on a daily basis.

78. **D.** The recommended caloric intake for a lactating mother is between 2,800 and 3,000 calories daily.

79. **C.** Lactogenesis is stimulated by an increase in luteotropic hormone and a decrease in estrogen and progesterone.

80. **C.** The nurse must serve in the role of resource person because the parents will ask questions not only about the new baby but other children at home.

81. **C.** The brassiere, to be effective in its purpose, should be worn 24 hours a day.

82. **C.** Propping of the infant's bottle also can lead to aspiration of the fluid.

83. **B.** The nurse should remember that the mother's expectations in regard to success are very high at this time and that the mother may never have seen anyone breast feed before.

84. **B.** The mother now recognizes that the child is no longer a part of her body and is now really a separate being.

85. **C.** Gerald Caplan uses this term in describing initial maternal behavior.

86. **B.** During this period of time, the child is not perceived as an extension of the mother. Thus, the mother cannot respond to his needs as quickly and assuredly as she would if seen as an extension of self.

87. **C.** Reva Rubin has described the three phases of emotional changes that take place during the postpartum period.

88. **D.** A mother's comfort and relaxed state provide a safe and secure environment for the infant.

89. **C.** These results occurred when mothers breast fed completely, that is, they did not supplement their infants with either the bottle or solid food.

90. **D.** It is not necessary for mothers to wash their nipples before each feeding because mother's milk contains lysozyme, an antibacterial enzyme.

91. **A.** This position is usually easiest at first for both mother and the nurse who may be assisting the mother.

92. **B.** There appears to be a trend toward breast feeding in the younger mothers who select the more natural way of feeding.

93. **B.** This organization was established in Illinois in 1956. The term "la leche" is taken from the Spanish language and means "the milk."

94. **B.** This procedure is suggested for use in the early nursing experience when the child is sleepy.

95. **D.** This decision is primarily up to the mother.

96. **D.** These mothers are not ready to assume maternal roles as early in the postpartum experience as other mothers.

97. **C.** These mothers *may* prefer that the child remain in the central nursery for at least the first day.

98. **A.** These mothers need a strong mother figure, and one who shows great affection toward the baby.

99. **B.** These feelings are normal, and much help can be given by the nurse regarding this.

100. **B.** These mothers display a strong attachment to the unborn child.

101. **D.** These mothers need much help in seeing that the baby is an individual and not a part of the woman.

102. **B.** Nonhuman mammalian mothers and human mothers follow an orderly progression of exploring their new infants. Fingertip contact is the first step in this progression.

103. **A.** The mother needs to know that although the initial onset of lactation may be delayed because the infant is not ready to nurse, the colostrum in her breasts will serve as nourishment until the child is ready to nurse well.

104. **B.** During the first week at home, she should restrict her stair climbing and stay on one floor.

105. **D.** The woman should abstain from coitus until she returns to the doctor for her six-week check.

106. **D.** All of the factors mentioned must be taken into consideration when thinking about the mother-infant relationship.

107. **A.** The condition remains localized or may spread to other organs and produce diverse clinical patterns.

108. **C.** The other organisms mentioned may also be responsible for disease conditions during the postpartum period, but the largest majority of conditions are due to streptococcal organisms.

109. **C.** Streptococcal organisms may be found in the vaginas of normal pregnant women. However, trauma and hemorrhage seem to be the determining factors in causing these organisms to become pathogenic.

110. **C.** Poor technique on the part of the medical and nursing staff is the main cause of puerperal fever.

111. **A.** Endometritis is a localized infection of the lining of the uterus.

112. **D.** Endometritis usually becomes evident about 48 to 72 hours following delivery.

113. **B.** In endometritis, the lochia is decreased in amount and may or may not have a foul odor, depending on the causative organisms.

114. **C.** However, if endometritis spreads to other organs, the disease may last for many weeks.

115. **B.** The most common localized infection is that of an infection of a repaired perineal laceration or episiotomy wound.

116. **C.** Ergonovine given at this time promotes uterine tone.

117. **C.** Thrombophlebitis is an infection of the vascular endothelium with clot formation attached to the vessel wall.

118. **C.** This is a severe complication of the postpartum period, usually occurring about the second week following delivery. The infection is usually caused by anaerobic streptococci.

119. **C.** Peritonitis can be a generalized or localized infection of the peritoneum.

120. **A.** Mayrhofer probably was the first person to see organisms causing puerperal fever.

121. **C.** Semmelweiss first determined that puerperal fever was transmitted from the dead, by contact from the physicians and students, to women in labor. He then determined that the fever could be transmitted from patient to patient by contact with contaminated articles or attendants.

122. **C.** Dr. Halsted was the first man to introduce sterile rubber gloves into the practive of medicine.

123. **B.** This paper was written in 1861. At this time, however, the actual cause of the disease was still unknown.

124. **D.** All of the factors mentioned are considered to be preventive measures.

125. **D.** The inflammation associated with a pelvic thrombophlebitis can extend, and the thrombus can also be broken into a mass of pus with small emboli breaking away.

126. **A.** This term may have been originated by those who believed that the inflammed leg actually contained milk. The skin over the area of swelling becomes tense and white. Also, lactation may cease when an acute febrile process is present.

127. **D.** With superficial femoral thrombophlebitis, anticoagulants are not usually administered. Only if the femoral thrombophlebitis is secondary to septic pelvic thrombophlebitis is the patient given antibiotics.

128. **B.** The causative agent in pelvic thrombophlebitis is usually anaerobic streptococcus.

129. **C.** The symptoms associated with femoral thrombophlebitis usually appear after the tenth postpartum day.

130. **B.** The uterine, ovarian, and hypogastric veins are involved in pelvic thrombophlebitis.

131. **C.** The clinical cause of pelvic peritonitis is like that of surgical peritonitis. Hiccoughs, nausea, and vomiting may be present.

132. **A.** Penicillin is effective against not only the hemolytic streptococcus but also the Welch bacillus and the staphylococcus.

133. **B.** If the insulin dosage is not reduced prior to delivery or immediately following, insulin shock will occur.

134. **D.** All of the factors predispose the breast for mastitis. Status of milk in a duct does not in itself cause infection but may injure the tissues and allow bacteria to enter more readily.

135. **C.** Puerperal mastitis may occur any time during lactation but usually occurs between the first and fourth week of the puerperium.

136. **C.** The engorgement per se does not cause the infection.

137. **D.** All of the factors mentioned will aid in the prevention of mastitis.

138. **D.** The infection is carried by the infant who has been exposed to the epidemic strain of the staphylococcus and is introduced through apparently normal lactiferous ducts in the breast.

139. **D.** All of the factors mentioned cause cystitis during the postpartum period.

140. **A.** The symptoms usually begin several days post partum. Temperature may rise to 100°F or to 101° F.

141. **D.** The mother should be observed for all of these as two early symptoms of congestive heart failure are edema and shortness of breath.

142. **A.** If the fundus is relaxed, the bleeding is probably caused by the failure of the muscle fibers to constrict the blood vessels.

143. **B.** To perform an internal bimanual compression, the right hand (gloved) is inserted into the vagina, and the anterior aspect of the uterus is massaged by the fingers of the right hand. At the same, the left hand is pressed deeply into the abdomen. Massage of the posterior aspect of the uterus is done with this hand.

144. **B.** However, replacement by blood is started promptly when bleeding becomes excessive.

145. **A.** An untreated gonorrheal infection can produce an inflammation of tubes, which may result in closure of the fimbriated opeings.

146. **B.** Vulvar hematomas are caused by the rupture of the subcutaneous veins of the vagina, which produces an effusion of blood into the connective tissue of the vulva and vaginal wall.

147. **D.** Vulvar hematomas may also occur within the episiotomy if a vein is pricked during repair.

148. **B.** RhoGAM contains the specific antibodies against Rh positive blood cells and thus suppress the development of the antibody.

149. **D.** All of these doctors were involved in the development of RhoGAM.

150. **C.** Although clinical trials were begun in 1964, widespread use of RhoGAM started about 1968.

151. **D.** It appears that when the placenta separates from the uterine wall, Rh positive fetal cells enter the maternal circulation, causing the mother to build up antibodies. The Rh antibodies in RhoGAM combine with the Rh antigen in the mother's bloodstream and neutralize it.

152. **C.** The usual dosage of RhoGAM is 200 to 300 µg given intramuscularly within 72 hours of delivery.

153. **D.** All of the points mentioned increase the possibility of fetomaternal hemorrhage and thus the possibility of immunization. Fetomaternal hemorrhage occurs primarily at the time of placental separation.

154. **B.** These mothers may have overwhelming physical or psychological needs that hinder the necessary emotional changes during the puerperium.

155. **D.** Subinvolution may also be caused by the presence of uterine fibroids.

156. **C.** Backache, a dragging sensation in the pelvis, and general poor health are also symptoms of subinvolution of the uterus.

157. **C.** Late (or delayed) postpartum hemorrhage occurs anywhere between the second and twenty-eighth day post partum.

158. **C.** Latent toxemia can occur during the postpartum period. A blood pressure of 130/90 or above can be significant.

159. **D.** All of these can be used to provide temporary relief of painful sutures.

160. **A.** The majority of postpartum hemorrhages occur during the first 12 hours.

161. **B.** Methergine may be administered to maintain uterine tone and prevent the accumulation of clots in the uterine cavity.

162. **B.** The incidence of vulvar and vaginal hematomas is about once in every 500 to 1,000 deliveries.

163. **B.** Agalactia rarely occurs. More frequently seen are cases in which the milk secretion is so scarce that there is insufficient quantity to supply the nourishment required by the infant. This condition is termed hypogalactia.

164. **C.** There are marked individual differences in the amount of milk secreted by the breast. This appears to be dependent on the degree of development of the glandular portions of the breasts.

165. **A.** If the breast-fed infant acquires this organism in the nursery, he may easily carry it to his mother.

166. **D.** All of the points mentioned indicate that the tension associated with the birth of the problem child is prolonged and intensified rather than being released in more customary ways.

167. **A.** The parents of a newborn do not know what is normal and what is not normal.

168. **D.** All of the factors mentioned contribute to the communication problems present when less-than-perfect babies are born.

169. **C.** Parents of premature infants also have great concern about the presence of deformities and mental retardation in their child.

170. **A.** The loss of their child will set off the grief process. The initial reaction will be one of disbelief and shock.

171. **C.** Upon learning that her child is less than perfect, the mother will create fantasies about the child's appearance. She must see the child in order to minimize her own fantasies.

172. **C.** Carunculae myrtiformes is the name given to the ragged edges of tissue that replace the hymenal ring after childbirth.

173. **D.** Diastasis is the name given to the separation of the recti muscles as a result of pregnancy.

174. **B.** Autolysis is the name given to the process by which involution takes place.

175. **A.** Bradycardia is the normal pulse rate during the early puerperium.

176. **C.** Agalactia is the absence of failure of the secretion of milk.

177. **D.** Galactagogue is the causing of the flow of milk.

178. **A.** Galactorrhea is an excessive flow of milk.

179. **B.** Galactopoiesis is the maintenance of milk.

180. **C.** Endometritis is a localized infection of the lining membrane of the uterus.

181. **A.** Endomyometritis is a localized infection of the inner muscular layer of the uterus.

182. **B.** Parametritis is an infection involving the peritoneum and broad ligaments.

183. **D.** Peritonitis is a generalized or local infection of the peritoneum.

184. **C.** A full bladder is considered to be one of the causes of postpartal hemorrhage.

185. **B.** Molding of the infant's head takes place during delivery and is caused by the intrauterine position or by the passage through the birth canal.

186. **D.** The woman must be told that she should increase her activity gradually.

187. **B.** The lochia normally is rubra for several days following the delivery.

188. **D.** An episiotomy eliminates a laceration, can be done in a direction of choice, avoids undue stretching of perineal musculature, and shortens the second stage of delivery.

189. **D.** After delivery and for about two days, the breasts continue to function much as they did during pregnancy. They secrete colostrum. After the first two days, the breast milk flows in and the breasts become larger, firmer, and more tender.

190. **C.** Immediately after delivery, the top of the fundus is often normally below the level of the umbilicus. It then rises to near the level of the umbilicus and remains there for several days. A firm fundus indicates that the uterine muscles are contracting as they should.

191. **B.** During the first several days post partum, the lochia will be primarily bright red because of the large amount of blood. The normal characteristic odor is fleshy and resembles that of menstrual blood.

192. **C.** Perineal sutures can cause considerable discomfort. Edema results both from the sutures and from excessive stretching of the tissues during delivery. Painful hemorrhoids are a common complaint during the puerperium. They may result from pressure and straining efforts during labor and delivery.

193. **B.** The temperature may rise to 101.4°F shortly after a long labor, but it should drop to normal within 24 hours. Sometimes the temperature may be slightly above normal during the first few days without other problems. The normal pulse

during the first seven to ten days may be 60 to 70 beats/min. It is believed that this puerperal brady-cardia is due to the decreased strain on the heart after birth of the infant and the reduction of the vascular bed with the contractions of the uterus.

194. **C.** Breast discomfort occurring during the first three or four days; the "initial breast engorge-ment" is due to venous engorgement.

195. **C.** Breast feeding should never be depended upon as a means of contraception. However, lac-tation has been shown to suppress ovulation for 75 days post partum in almost 100% of mothers who did not supplement their infants with bottle or solid food.

196. **D.** The protein requirement is increased by 10 g (over nonpregnant requirements) during preg-nancy and by 2 g (over nonpregnant requirements) during the period of lactation.

197. **A.** The size of the breasts is largely due to the amount of fatty tissue they contain and, therefore, is not indicative of ability to produce milk.

198. **C.** Ideally, Mrs. Lancaster should have been admitted 24 hours prior to surgery. She would have then received the same type of preparation as any preoperative patient. However, since she came into the hospital in labor, she will probably not receive an enema. She will not be given mor-phine prior to surgery, as any narcotic can depress the baby's respirations. She will also have a type and cross match done for several pints of blood.

199. **B.** The low segment cesarean section is usually considered to be the section of coice. In this type of surgery there is less danger of infection or hemorrhage, better healing of the wound, and less chance of subsequent rupture of the uterus in fu-ture pregnancies.

200. **B.** The higher fetal mortality rate is attributed to pre-existing complications in the mother that may lead to problems in the infant.

201. **D.** The most serious complications following a cesarean section are hemorrhage and infection. However, ileus and acute dilatation of the stomach may also occur following abdominal sur-gery of this type.

202. **D.** All of the orders mentioned could appear on Mrs. Lancaster's chart.

203. **B.** A postspinal headache occurs as a result of leakage of spinal fluid at the puncture site with a reduction of spinal fluid pressure.

204. **D.** It is a routine practice to send the infant born by cesarean section to the nursery almost im-mediately after birth. The mother may have had a fleeting look at the infant. However, before she can rest comfortably she must see for herself that her child is doing well.

205. **B.** Internal hemorrhage could be suspected if there was an increase in the pulse and respiratory rates and a drop in the blood pressure. Re-member, however, a drop in the blood pressure could be the result of some anesthetic drugs.

206. **B.** Mrs. Lancaster may have trouble regaining control of her body functioning because of the sur-gery itself.

207. **C.** There is no reason why Mrs. lancaster cannot breast feed her infant. She may need additional help during the feeding periods, however, because of her difficulty in moving about confortably.

208. **B.** Mrs. Lancaster may have increased anxiety regarding her abdominal incision during the post-partal period. The increased amount of lochia that results following ambulation may be seen as the onset of increased bleeding rather than the normal flow.

209. **C.** The woman who does not deliver her baby vaginally may feel that she did not fulfill her role as a woman.

210. **C.** Large amounts of ice water or iced drinks may increase the amount of flatus following sur-gery.

211. **B.** Although Mrs. Lancaster had been prepared for a cesarean section at term, the suddenness of the surgery at the thirty-eighth week of pregnancy and the labor that followed may not have given her ample chance to prepare psychologically for her new son. Mrs. Lancaster may have felt that she was a participant in the birth process because she was awake when the child was born.

212. **C.** Providing that Mrs. Lancaster's recovery phase is not a complicated one, she will probably go home on the eighth to the tenth postpartum day.

213. **B.** Mrs. Lancaster will probably be asked to see her doctor in two weeks following hospital dis-charge to make sure that the incision is healing correctly and to check for further complica-tions.

CHAPTER 7

The Newborn

The nurse who works in the newborn nursery has the opportunity to play a variety of roles with both the infant and its mother.

In this chapter on the newborn infant are questions relating to the early care of both the normal and the abnormal child. Of particular significance here is material pertaining to premature and low-birth-weight infants.

The situational questions in this chapter test your general knowledge regarding the necessary care that should be given to the newborn baby in both the delivery room and the nursery.

Directions: Each of the questions or incomplete statements below is followed by four suggested answers or completions. Select the BEST answer in each case.

1. Extrauterine life is dependent upon adequate maturation of the lungs. This may be present by what week of gestation?
   A. 22 weeks
   B. 24 weeks
   C. 26 weeks
   D. 28 weeks   (8:536−7)

2. Which of the following structures first begins to function immediately after the birth of the baby?
   A. circulatory system
   B. respiratory system
   C. temperature regulating system
   D. urinary system   (8:540)

3. Surfactant is
   A. a natural coating on the skin at birth
   B. a liquid found in the stomach at birth
   C. a natural coating on the alveolar surface of the lungs at birth
   D. a liquid found in the small intestines at birth   (7:149)

4. The main component of surfactant is
   A. sphingomyelin
   B. lecithin
   C. phospholipids
   D. none of the above   (6:478)

5. The production of surfactant in the newborn can be decreased in which of the following situations?
   A. administration of oxygen at extremely high pressure
   B. chilling of the newborn
   C. in the immature baby
   D. all of the above   (3:529−30)

6. The first step in the immediate care of the newborn baby is to
   A. appraise the infant by the Apgar score
   B. provide warmth
   C. suction secretions to open airway
   D. provide intermittent positive pressure if there is no spontaneous respiratory movement   (4:341)

7. It is believed that the onset of respiration in the newborn is influenced by
   A. the varying degrees of asphyxia present in all infants at birth
   B. the chemical changes in the blood that result from the asphyxia

C. physical stimulation resulting from the birth process

D. all of the above (8:540)

8. Postponing the clamping of the umbilical cord until it stops pulsating may result in

A. an increased amount of iron to the infant

B. mild pulmonary edema

C. incidence of pulmonary rales and transient cyanosis

D. all of the above (3:532-3)

9. An Apgar score of 9 indicates that the baby is

A. in danger of dying

B. having a great deal of respiratory difficulty

C. in good condition

D. cyanotic and needs more oxygen (4:343)

10. Which one of the following would indicate that a newborn child rated an Apgar score of 3 on reflex irritability?

A. child responds to a slap on the sole of the foot with a cry

B. child responds with a cough or sneeze when a catheter is placed just inside its nose

C. child responds to attempts to extend its arm or leg with resistance

D. none of the above (8:394)

11. Silver nitrate 1% is instilled into the eyes of the newborn as a preventive measure against

A. ophthalmia neonatorum

B. spirochetal infection

C. streptococcal infection

D. icterus neonatorum (4:599-600)

12. Vitamin K, frequently administered to infants at birth,

A. prepares the infant for blood loss

B. aids in the clotting process

C. prevents destruction of red blood cells by strengthening the cell wall

D. prevents infection (4:591)

13. Which of the following contribute to the relative instability of body temperatures in the newborn?

A. immature mechanisms of sweating and shivering

B. large body surfaces in relation to the body mass

C. meager amount of subcutaneous fat

D. all of the above (3:533)

14. The period during which fetal circulation undergoes conversion to adult circulation is termed

A. period of newborn stress

B. period of neonatal adjustment

C. period of transitional circulation

D. none of the above (8:542)

15. Which of the following leads to the establishment of the adult pattern of circulation?

A. closure of the foramen ovule

B. closure of the ductus arteriosus

C. obliteration of umbilical vessls

D. all of the above (3:531)

16. The foramen ovule and ductus arteriosus anatomically close

A. completely, immediately after the birth of the baby

B. completely, within minutes after birth

C. within hours after birth

D. within weeks or months after birth (8:541-2)

17. The first four-week period following birth of an infant is usually termed the

A. neonatal period

B. prenatal period

C. infant period

D. none of the above (8:535)

18. The average birth weight of a full-term Caucasian baby is

A. 7 lb

B. 7 lb, 2 oz

C. 7 lb, 4 oz

D. 7 lb, 8 oz (8:556)

19. The average length of the full-term infant is approximately

A. 18 in.

B. 18.5 in.

C. 19 in.

D. 19.5 in. (8:558)

20. A physical assessment of the newborn infant should begin by observing the child

A. in the resting posture

B. in the crying posture

C. in the nursing posture

D. none of the above (1:237)

21. The frog position is normal in

A. babies born in vertex position

B. babies born in breech position

C.   all newborns
D.   none of the above   (1:237)

22.   The head of the newborn constitutes how much of the total body?

A.   one eighth
B.   one fourth
C.   one third
D.   one tenth   (3:551)

23.   Molding is

A.   the shaping of the baby's head as the child moves through the birth canal
B.   the shaping of the baby's head, which is dependent upon the child's position during the early weeks of extrauterine life
C.   the shaping of the baby's head during a cesarean section
D.   none of the above   (8:559)

24.   At birth the average circumference of the full-term baby's head ranges from

A.   31 to 36 cm
B.   28 to 30 cm
C.   35 to 40 cm
D.   none of the above   (8:562)

25.   The white substance that may be present within the folds of the labia is called

A.   vernix
B.   smegma
C.   lanugo
D.   none of the above   (6:395)

26.   Which one of the following glands is active immediately following birth?

A.   sweat glands
B.   sebaceous glands
C.   lacrimal glands
D.   none of the above   (8:574)

27.   Small flat hemangiomas or "stork bites" seen in the newborn may be expected to

A.   become much lighter in color and/or disappear during infancy
B.   become darker and grow as the child grows
C.   remain about the same throughout the child's life
D.   become lighter in color in several weeks   (1:17–8)

28.   The maturity of the newborn can be estimated by the number and kind of creases found

A.   on the buttock area
B.   on the palms of the hand
C.   on the soles of the feet
D.   all of the above   (7:148)

29.   The posterior fontanel is palpated as an opening in the skull. It is formed by the

A.   frontal and parietal bones
B.   parietal and occipital bones
C.   temporal and frontal bones
D.   frontal and occipital bones (8:562)

30.   Cephalhematoma is

A.   an edematous swelling of the soft tissue of the scalp, present immediately after birth
B.   a collection of blood between the periosteum and skull bone, present several hours after birth
C.   a collection of blood anywhere in the cranial vault, occurring after birth
D.   none of the above   (4:597)

31.   Another name for the blueness of the hands and feet present in the newborn during the first 24 hours of life is

A.   acromion
B.   acrocyanosis
C.   acromegalic
D.   acromicria   (5:187)

32.   Which of the following are not normally seen in the newborn infant?

A.   lanugo
B.   milia
C.   mongolian spots
D.   none of the above   (5:191)

33.   Which one of the following is not considered abnormal during the early newborn period?

A.   pemphigus neonatorum
B.   erythema toxicum neonatorum
C.   miliaria
D.   none of the above   (3:553)

34.   The iris of the eye may not assume its permanent color until the child is about

A.   3 months old
B.   6 months old
C.   9 months old
D.   12 months old   (7:153)

35. During the earliest days of life, the child can
    A. not see at all
    B. distinguish light from dark
    C. see and discriminate patterns and colors
    D. none of the above (3:566)

36. Acute hearing in the newborn
    A. is not possible until there is further physical maturation of the ears and nerve tracts
    B. is present at birth
    C. occurs gradually after aeration of eustachian tubes and discharge of mucus from the middle ear
    D. all of the above (4:405)

37. The average respiratory rate of the newborn infant is approximately
    A. 30/min
    B. 40/min
    C. 50/min
    D. 60/min (8:541)

38. The average pulse rate of the newborn infant is
    A. 100 to 120 beats/min
    B. 120 to 140 beats/min
    C. 80 to 100 beats/min
    D. 130 to 150 beats/min (8:544)

39. The average number of red blood cells in the normal newborn infant at birth is
    A. 5 million per cubic mm
    B. 4 million per cubic mm
    C. 6 million per cubic mm
    D. 7 million per cubic mm (8:544)

40. The total number of white blood cells in the normal newborn is
    A. 5,000 to 15,000 cells/μL
    B. 10,000 to 30,000 cells/μL
    C. 15,000 to 45,000 cells/μL
    D. 20,000 to 60,000 cells/μL (4:401)

41. The newborn's blood accounts for what percentage of its total body weight?
    A. 3%
    B. 5%
    C. 8%
    D. 10% (6:401)

42. Meconium, the first stools of the newborn, contains
    A. lanugo and vernix caseosa
    B. digestive secretions and mucus

C. bile pigments
D. all of the above (8:564)

43. Transitional stools are
    A. greenish-black
    B. greenish-brown
    C. greenish-yellow
    D. brownish-yellow (8:565)

44. During the first day of life, the approximate amount of urine voided by the newborn is
    A. 1 to 2 oz
    B. 3 to 4 oz
    C. 4 to 5 oz
    D. 5 to 6 oz (8:567)

45. Which of the following conditions in the newborn baby is the result of a hormonal factor?
    A. harlequin color changes
    B. engorged breasts
    C. thrush
    D. none of the above (4:408)

46. Following birth, approximately how long does it take for the infant's temperature to return to its normal state?
    A. 2 hours
    B. 8 hours
    C. 10 hours
    D. 12 hours (4:400)

47. What percentage of the newborn's weight is extracellular water?
    A. 15 to 20%
    B. 30 to 40%
    C. 70 to 75%
    D. none of the above (6:393)

48. The normal bleeding time for the infant at birth is
    A. half a minute
    B. one minute
    C. two minutes
    D. four minutes (6:405)

49. The normal coagulation time for the infant at birth is
    A. one minute
    B. two minutes
    C. three minutes
    D. four minutes (6:405)

50. Which of the following conditions would be contraindications for circumcision?
    1. abnormal bleeding time
    2. cephalo hematoma

3. vomiting
4. nevus flammeus
5. skin eruptions

   A. 1, 3, 5
   B. 1, 2, 4, 5
   C. 2, 4
   D. all of the above   (6:405)

51. The prothrombin level is highest

   A. at birth
   B. within 24 hours
   C. within 48 hours
   D. none of the above   (6:405)

52. The hemoglobin level of the newborn at birth measures from

   A. 12 to 17 g/dL of blood
   B. 13 to 18 g/dL of blood
   C. 14 to 19 g/dL of blood
   D. 15 to 20 g/dL of blood   (8:544−5)

53. Which of the following bilirubin rates in the newborn infant is considered to be of a pathologic nature?

   A. above 9 mg/dL
   B. above 11 mg/dL
   C. above 13 mg/dL
   D. above 16 mg/dL   (8:546)

54. During the first few days of life it can be expected that the newborn baby will lose approximately

   A. 1 to 5% of birth weight
   B. 5 to 10% of birth weight
   C. 10 to 15% of birth weight
   D. none of the above   (8:556)

55. The capacity of the normal newborn's stomach has been estimated to be

   A. 25 to 35 cc
   B. 30 to 40 cc
   C. 40 to 50 cc
   D. 50 to 60 cc   (4:403)

56. Which of the following reflexes is termed a "protective reflex"?

   A. yawning
   B. stepping
   C. rooting
   D. gagging   (4:402)

57. Which of the following is functioning at a minimum level at birth in the normal neonate?

   A. moro reflex
   B. gastric secretions

   C. salivary secretions
   D. stepping reflex   (8:563)

58. The tonic neck reflex normally

   A. is never present at birth
   B. is always present at birth
   C. is sometimes present at birth
   D. none of the above   (1:247)

59. The most effective way of eliciting the moro reflex is by placing the child on its back in the crib, then supporting trunk with one hand, and head and neck with the other hand and then

   A. releasing hold on trunk
   B. releasing hold on head and neck
   C. releasing both hands, allowing child to fall back on the mattress of the crib
   D. none of the above   (1:251−2)

60. The moro reflex is normally absent

   A. immediately after birth
   B. 24 hours after birth
   C. by the time of the child's discharge from the hospital
   D. four to five months after birth   (8:582)

61. Several newborn reflexes can be grouped together because they have a common purpose. Which one of the following groupings illustrates the feeding reflexes?

   A. moro, rooting, dancing
   B. sneezing, coughing, blinking
   C. sucking, rooting, swallowing
   D. tonic neck, moro, grasping   (8:584−5)

62. The following characteristics are normal in newborns

   1. a receding chin
   2. a skin erythema, loose stool
   3. mongolian spots, milia
   4. head circumference larger than chest

   A. 1
   B. 2, 3
   C. 1, 3
   D. 1, 3, 4   (8:559−623, 573−4)

63. Nevi vasculosi are

   A. purple capillary hemangiomas
   B. dark blue areas distributed over the lumbar, sacral, and gluteal regions
   C. bright or dark red capillary hemangiomas
   D. small, reddened areas produced by capillary hemangiomas   (6:392)

64. The name given to the fold of tissue that connects the tongue to the floor of the mouth and occasionally causes nursing problems for the child is
    A. masseter muscle
    B. frenulum linguae
    C. adenoid tissue
    D. none of the above   (6:393—4)

65. The lacrimal glands begin to function
    A. during the last months of fetal life
    B. shortly after birth
    C. within two to six weeks of life
    D. about eight weeks after birth   (6:395)

66. What substance in human breast milk inhibits the activity of glucuronyl transferase?
    A. pregnanediol
    B. serum albumin
    C. sugar
    D. none of the above   (6:402)

67. Which of the following is *not* associated with physiologic jaundice in the normal newborn?
    A. Coombs' test positive
    B. jaundice after about 36 hours
    C. bilirubin level 5 to 7 mg/dL on third day
    D. jaundice disappears before fourteenth day of age   (6:402)

68. Physiologic jaundice in the newborn is caused by
    A. polycythemia present in the normal newborn
    B. immature liver functioning
    C. both A and B
    D. neither A nor B   (6:402)

69. Physiologic jaundice
    1. indicates a deficiency in blood coagulation ability
    2. is associated with dehydration caused by a low fluid intake the first few days of life
    3. results from a breakdown of red blood cells, which then increase the level of serum bilirubin
    4. is in part due to immature functioning ability of the liver of the neonate
    5. is indicated by a bilirubin level above 12 mg/dL of blood
    A. 3, 4
    B. 3, 4, 5
    C. 1, 2, 3
    D. 2, 3, 4   (6:402)

70. What is the name of the enzyme that brings about the conversion of the bilirubin from an insoluble to a soluble form in the newborn?
    A. cytolytic
    B. hyaluronidase
    C. proleolytic
    D. glucuronyl transferase   (6:402)

71. Which of the following are characteristic of the early stools of the breast-fed infant?
    1. feces soft
    2. low pH of 5 to 6
    3. greenish yellow
    4. strong odor caused by putrefative bacteria
    5. less frequent movements
    A. 1, 3, 5
    B. 1, 2, 3
    C. 2, 3, 4
    D. all of the above   (6:403)

72. The high lactose content in breast milk is converted into lactic acid by which of the following substances?
    A. hydrochloric acid
    B. *Lactobacillus bifidus*
    C. pepsin
    D. rennin   (6:403)

73. A high lactose content in breast milk is considered to be an advantage because
    A. it aids in increasing the mineral content of the child's bones
    B. it produces an acid medium in the lower gastrointestinal tract
    C. it encourages the production of riboflavin and pyridoxine in the intestines
    D. all of the above   (6:411—2)

74. The protein found in the newborn's feeding is acted upon by
    A. gastric chemistry
    B. pancreatic secretions
    C. intestinal secretions
    D. all of the above   (6:403)

75. The most usual treatment for meconium plug syndrome is
    A. use of suppositories
    B. use of a mild cathartic
    C. increased fluid intake
    D. digital examination   (6:404)

76. The bowel movements that occur following each feeding are the result of
    A. insufficient burping of the child
    B. too rapid feeding
    C. gastrocolic reflex
    D. excessive amount of sugar in the formula (6:404)

77. The most important treatment for miliaria is
    A. antibiotics
    B. antielongic formula
    C. reduction in amount of clothing
    D. all of the above (1:21)

78. Seborrheic dermatitis is usually seen
    A. behind the ears or behind the knees
    B. on the feet and palms
    C. on the forehead, cheeks, neck, and chest
    D. none of the above (1:22)

79. The usual treatment for seborrheic dermatitis is
    A. daily washing with soap and water
    B. antibiotics
    C. change in the detergent used for the infant's clothing and bedding
    D. none of the above (1:22)

80. Which of the following statements best describes common diaper rash?
    A. bright red, raised, draining papules
    B. red, macular, diffuse rash
    C. mild erythematous nonraised areas
    D. none of the above (1:22)

81. Which of the following are normally found in the mouth of the newborn?
    A. Epstein's pearls
    B. Koplik spots
    C. Bednar's aphthae
    D. all of the above (1:105−6)

82. Which of the following can be considered to be predisposing factors in functional vomiting in the newborn?
    1. propping of the bottle
    2. too large openings in nipple
    3. too rapid feeding
    4. lack of sufficient "bubbling" of the infant
    5. formula too dilute
    A. 1, 3, 5
    B. 2, 3, 4, 5
    C. none of the above
    D. all of the above (6:424)

83. The protein requirement for the newborn can be fulfilled by what quantity of formula per day?
    A. 1 oz/lb of body weight
    B. ½ oz/lb of body weight
    C. 2 oz/lb of body weight
    D. none of the above (6:421)

84. What is the necessary iron intake for the newborn infant?
    A. 0.5 to 1 mg/kg of body weight
    B. 1 to 2 mg/kg of body weight
    C. 2 to 3 mg/kg of body weight
    D. 3 to 4 mg/kg of body weight (6:422)

85. Which of the following signs would indicate that an infant needs to have its formula strengthened?
    1. shows a steady gain in weight
    2. cries an hour or so following a feeding
    3. shows good muscle tone during his activity
    4. takes large amounts of formula at frequent intervals
    5. shows a moderate amount of subcutaneous fat
    A. 1, 3, 5
    B. 2, 4
    C. none of the above
    D. all of the above (6:424)

86. Breast milk is distinguished from colostrum by
    1. a bluish-white rather than yellow fluid
    2. increased quantity of the fluid
    3. the accompanying sensations of heavy, full breasts
    4. a higher protein and lower carbohydrate content
    A. 1, 2
    B. 1, 2, 3
    C. 2, 3, 4
    D. 1, 2, 3, 4 (8:617)

87. The infant's caloric needs are usually based on
    A. weight gain
    B. well-being
    C. satiety
    D. all of the above (4:401)

88. The infant's basal metabolism per kilogram of body weight is
    A. lower than that of an adult
    B. same as that of an adult

C.   higher than that of an adult
D.   none of the above   (4:400)

89.   Caloric intake in the newborn is necessary to

A.   provide energy for the metabolic needs
B.   provide for rapid growth
C.   provide for daily increasing activity
D.   all of the above   (8:615)

90.   Once the newborn baby has passed the first few days of life his daily caloric needs are

A.   about 90 to 100 calories per kg of body weight
B.   about 100 to 110 calories per kg of body weight
C.   about 110 to 120 calories per kg of body weight
D.   about 120 to 130 calories per kg of body weight   (4:401)

91.   By the time the baby is 7 to 10 days old, his caloric needs are

A.   100 to 120 calories per kg of body weight
B.   110 to 130 calories per kg of body weight
C.   120 to 140 calories per kg of body weight
D.   140 to 160 calories per kg of body weight   (8:615)

92.   Transitory fever in the newborn is caused by

A.   diarrhea
B.   infection
C.   fever of unknown origin
D.   imbalance between fluid loss and fluid intake   (4:401)

93.   Transitory fever of the newborn is most frequently found in infants who

A.   do not take their feedings well
B.   are excessively large
C.   are excessively small
D.   none of the above   (4:401)

94.   Self-regulating (self-demand) feeding schedule means

A.   feeding the baby on a regular schedule and giving it all it will take
B.   feeding the baby every time it cries and giving it all it desires
C.   feeding the baby when it is hungry and giving it all that it desires
D.   none of the above   (8:614)

95.   The normal newborn's need for fluid intake is

A.   greater than that of an adult
B.   lesser than that of an adult
C.   same as that of an adult
D.   none of the above   (8:615)

96.   The infant's requirement for fluid intake per 24 hours is

A.   100 to 150 mL per kg of body weight
B.   125 to 175 mL per kg of body weight
C.   150 to 200 mL per kg of body weight
D.   175 to 225 mL per kg of body weight   (8:616)

97.   What is the minimal 24-hour water requirement for a normal full-term newborn?

A.   30 to 45 mL per kg of body weight
B.   45 to 60 mL per kg of body weight
C.   60 to 75 mL per kg of body weight
D.   75 to 90 mL per kg of body weight   (8:616)

98.   The method of choice in infant feeding is influenced by

A.   mores of a society
B.   cultural setting
C.   previous experiences and attitudes
D.   all of the above   (5:194)

99.   The reservoir within the breast for human milk is called

A.   tubercles of Montgomery
B.   lactiferous sinus
C.   alveoli
D.   areolae   (8:617)

100.   The production of colostrum starts

A.   after the third month of pregnancy
B.   after the sixth month of pregnancy
C.   after the eighth month of pregnancy
D.   immediately after delivery of the infant   (8:117)

101.   Responding to the newborn when he cries will

A.   spoil the child
B.   condition the child to cry more often
C.   decrease the amount of crying the child does and also make him less demanding
D.   none of the above   (7:158)

102.   A new mother asks how she will know when her baby is hungry. Which of the following responses would be most appropriate for the nurse to make?

A. crying usually indicates hunger
B. feed the baby whenever it is awake
C. it will cry, fret, and suck on anything coming in contact with its lips
D. offer it water first; if it refuses the water, then feed it (8:589)

103. The term "asphyxia neonatorum" refers to a condition
A. experienced by all newborn babies during delivery
B. in which the newborn's respirations are not established within the first minute of life
C. experienced by all newborn babies until the adult circulation pattern has been established
D. none of the above (5:304—5)

104. Failure of the infant to breathe at birth is usually caused by
A. intrauterine hypoxia
B. drugs
C. central nervous system trauma
D. all of the above (8:696)

105. Hyaline membrane disease is *most* frequently seen in infants
A. weighing between 1,000 and 1,500 g
B. of diabetic mothers
C. of mothers who experienced antepartal vaginal bleeding
D. weighing less than 2,500 g (4:595)

106. Which of the following theories regarding the cause of hyaline membrane disease has been suggested?
A. there is an alteration of the fibrinolytic enzyme in the lungs or blood, which leads to the proliferation of a protein exudate
B. there is an alteration in, or an absence of, pulmonary surfactant, which reduces alveolar ventilation and promotes atelectasis
C. there is pulmonary hypofusion rather than surfactant deficiency
D. all of the above (4:594)

107. Visually, the first symptom of hyaline membrane disease is
A. sternal and subcostal retractions
B. rapid respirations
C. low body temperature
D. expiratory grunting (4:595)

108. Intracranial hemorrhage in the newborn occurs most often following
A. normal labors
B. cesarean sections
C. induced labors
D. prolonged labors (4:597)

109. Symptoms such as cyanosis, vomiting, listlessness, and poor sucking are indicative of
A. cerebral irritation
B. respiratory distress
C. congenital heart disease
D. all of the above (8:760—1)

110. The baby who has cerebral injury may have
A. a high-pitched cry
B. an anxious expression
C. pale, clammy skin
D. all of the above (8:761)

111. The moro reflex in the baby with cerebral hemorrhage
A. is not present at birth
B. is present at birth
C. is not present after 24 hours
D. none of the above (8:761)

112. The usual treatment for a baby with cerebral injury is primarily based on
A. stimulation of the infant
B. giving of large amounts of fluid
C. rest and quiet
D. none of the above (8:761)

113. The infant who may have a cerebral injury should be in the crib
A. with head lowered
B. with head raised
C. with head and feet level
D. on his right side (4:598)

114. Which of the following will probably be used in the treatment of the baby with cerebral injury?
A. incubator
B. vitamin K
C. phenobarbital
D. all of the above (8:761—2)

115. Which of the following is a common sequela of permanent cerebral damage?
A. blindness
B. cerebral palsy
C. deformity of the hand
D. none of the above (8:762)

116. Which of the following techniques is basically most important in preventing infections in the newborn nursery?

    A. autoclaving all clothing and linen for babies
    B. obtaining nose and throat cultures for nursery personnel
    C. providing written policies concerning asepsis
    D. handwashing before each contact with an infant (4:408—9)

117. Thrush in the neonate is caused by

    A. *Candida albicans*
    B. *Treponema pallidum*
    C. *Herpesvirus hominis*
    D. *Neisseria gonorrhoeae* (4:601)

118. Gonorrheal conjunctivitis can be transmitted to the newborn

    A. during the birth process
    B. by the contaminated hands of nurses and doctors
    C. by contaminated articles
    D. all of the above (4:599)

119. Which one of the following statements best describes the early signs of gonorrheal conjunctivitis?

    A. edema and redness of the eyelids, purulent discharges lasting 24 to 48 hours
    B. edema and redness of the eyelids and conjunctiva, copious purulent discharge that begins within the second or third day after birth
    C. edema and redness of the eyelids, purulent discharge which begins after the fifth to seventh day of life
    D. none of the above (8:741—2)

120. Congenital syphilis is transmitted from the mother to the child

    A. sometime during the first month of pregnancy
    B. sometime during the second and third months of pregnancy
    C. sometime during the fifth month of pregnancy and end of pregnancy
    D. at birth (8:742)

121. Congenital syphilis can best be detected in the infant by

    A. testing the blood of the mother immediately prior to the birth of the child
    B. physical assessment of the child at birth
    C. testing the blood of the child immediately following birth
    D. testing the blood of the child once a month or more often over a period of several months (8:743)

122. Hemolytic disease of the newborn is caused by

    A. inborn errors of metabolism
    B. blood-group incompatibility between mother and child
    C. deficiency of coagulation factors depending upon vitamin K
    D. sex-linked recessive mendelian tract (3:790)

123. Which of the following hemolytic diseases is considered to be the most serious disease for the newborn?

    A. Rh incompatibility
    B. A incompatibility
    C. hyperbilirubinemia
    D. B incompatibility (3:790)

124. The classical sign(s) of hemolytic disease of newborns are

    A. anemia
    B. jaundice
    C. edema
    D. all of the above (8:727)

125. Which one of the following have been found useful in the prevention of erythroblastosis fetalis?

    A. vitamin K
    B. vitamin E
    C. RhoGAM
    D. vitamin C (2:298—9)

126. When an Rh positive man and an Rh negative woman plan to have children, will an incompatibility for Rh factor always result?

    A. yes, because the child will be Rh negative and, as a result, develop antibodies to the father's Rh positive blood
    B. no, because the father, although he possesses Rh positive blood, may be heterozygous for Rh factor
    C. yes, because the child will develop Rh antibodies to the mother's blood
    D. no, because the mother will not develop antibodies to the fetus' blood (2:296)

127. The direct Coombs' test measures

    A. surfactant levels in the fetus
    B. fibrinogen levels in the fetus

C. estriol levels in the mother

D. blood agglutination in the baby caused by Rh factor (8:730)

128. Which of the following maternal complications gives rise to a newborn infant who has hypoglycemia?

A. toxemia
B. diabetes
C. rubella
D. erythroblastosis (8:717)

129. Infants of diabetic mothers are highly susceptible to

A. erythroblastosis
B. respiratory distress syndrome (hyaline membrane disease)
C. retrolental fibroplasia
D. excitability and tremors (4:559)

130. Which of the following factors may contribute to congenital malformations?

A. maternal rubella
B. maternal age
C. radiation exposure during early pregnancy
D. all of the above (8:744)

131. Hydrocephalus is a condition in the newborn whereby

A. a large part of cerebral hemispheres is lacking
B. there is an accumulation of fluid in the intracranial cavity
C. there is a developmental defect in the closure of the long spinal canal
D. none of the above (4:503)

132. One of the most usual symptoms associated with esophageal atresia is

A. vomiting
B. fever
C. asphyxia
D. difficulty in swallowing (8:749)

133. The incidence of cleft lip and cleft palate is about one in every

A. 300 births
B. 400 births
C. 600 births
D. 800 births (2:273)

134. Cleft palate with or without the associated cleft lip is seen

A. more frequently in male infants
B. more frequently in female infants
C. in equal distribution between male and female infants
D. none of the above (3:820)

135. Cleft lips and cleft palates are the result of

A. incomplete fusion of maxillary or premaxillary processes during the fifth to eighth week of intrauterine life
B. incomplete fusion of the palatal processes during the twelfth week of intrauterine life
C. both A and B
D. none of the above (3:820)

136. The major problems associated with cleft palates during the early days of life are

A. immature temperature regulation
B. blood loss and infection
C. feeding and infection
D. transitory fever (8:748)

137. A cleft lip is

A. a congenital fissure in the upper lip
B. a fissure that may be unilateral or bilateral
C. a fissure that may vary from a slight notch to a complete separation extending into the nostril
D. all of the above (8:748)

138. Which one of the following chromosomal patterns is present in Down's syndrome?

A. trisomy 13-15
B. trisomy 17-18
C. trisomy 18-19
D. trisomy 21-22 (4:610)

139. The physical characteristics of Down's syndrome include

A. small cranium with sloping forehead; eyes are unusually small or have cataracts or iris defects; bulbous nose; hands and feet often grossly deformed
B. small cranium with flat occiput; eyes are set wide apart with lateral upward slope; short nose with flat bridge; hands are short and thick with simian creases on palmar surfaces
C. small cranium with prominent occiput; eyes usually normal; small mouth; malformed hands with clenched fists and index finger overlapping third finger
D. none of the above (8:756)

140. The incidence of Down's syndrome is approximately
    A. 0.5 in 1,000 births
    B. 1.0 in 1,000 births
    C. 1.5 in 1,000 births
    D. 2.0 in 1,000 births   (4:610)

141. A premature infant by the newest criteria is one who
    A. weighs 2,500 g or less at birth
    B. is born prior to the thirty-seventh week of gestation
    C. is born prior to the fortieth week of gestation
    D. none of the above   (3:795)

142. A low-birth-weight baby is one who
    A. weighs 1,500 g or less at birth
    B. weighs 2,500 g or less at birth
    C. weighs 3,000 g or less at birth
    D. none of the above   (3:795)

143. Which of the following contribute to death in the immature baby?
    A. respiratory problems
    B. intracranial hemorrhage
    C. infection
    D. all of the above   (8:670)

144. Which of the following have been known to contribute to prematurity?
    A. fetal conditions
    B. maternal factors
    C. placental factors
    D. all of the above   (4:555)

145. Which of the following features are characteristic of the premature infant?
    A. the skin is transparent and covered with lanugo
    B. respirations are shallow and irregular
    C. the skull is round with large fontanels
    D. all of the above   (4:563)

146. Recent studies indicate that premature infants do well when the relative humidity in the incubator is kept between
    A. 40 and 60%
    B. 55 and 65%
    C. 65 and 75%
    D. 75 and 85%   (6:471)

147. The infant with RDS
    A. has a greater tendency to develop hyperbilirubinemia
    B. has a lesser tendency to develop hyperbilirubinemia

    C. has about the same chance of developing hyperbilirubinemia as the full-term infant
    D. none of the above   (6:483)

148. Inborn errors of metabolism occur because of
    A. alteration of tissues during intrauterine development
    B. mutation in a molecule of the gene
    C. unknown reasons
    D. none of the above   (3:210)

149. PKU is a disorder in which there is an absence of
    A. the decarboxylase enzyme
    B. phenylalamine hydroxylase
    C. galactose 1-phosphate uridyl transferase
    D. none of the above   (3:211)

150. Infants with PKU are usually
    A. mildly retarded at birth
    B. moderately retarded at birth
    C. severely retarded at birth
    D. normal at birth   (3:211)

151. A positive diagnosis of PKU can be made when the phenylalanine level in the blood is
    A. less than 1 to 3 mg/dL of blood
    B. about 3 to 6 mg/dL of blood
    C. about 8 or more mg/dL of blood
    D. none of the above   (4:614)

152. The treatment of PKU consists of providing a dietary intake that has
    A. complete absence of protein
    B. large amounts of protein
    C. normal amounts of protein and absence of galactose
    D. adequate protein for growth and development only   (2:472)

153. Phenylketonuria can be most advantageously diagnosed from
    A. newborn's urine during the first 24 hours of life
    B. newborn's urine during the fourth day of life
    C. newborn's blood during the second day of life
    D. none of the above   (4:614)

154. Peripheral nerve injuries may occur
    A. during intrauterine life
    B. during birth

C. immediately after birth
D. none of the above   (8:758)

155. The most common injury occurring during labor and delivery is

A. brachial palsy
B. facial paralysis
C. diaphragmatic paralysis
D. none of the above   (8:758)

156. Erb-Duchenne Paralysis (Bells) is usually the result of

A. pressure against the facial nerve
B. injury to the fifth and sixth cervical nerves
C. injury to the seventh and eighth cervical nerves
D. injury to the phrenic nerve   (8:759)

157. The bone most commonly fractured during delivery is the

A. jaw
B. cervical spine
C. clavicle
D. femur   (8:758)

158. Pyloric stenosis is caused by

A. a membrane that covers the anus
B. a protrusion of the abdominal viscera
C. a constriction of the lumen of the pyloric opening
D. a failure of union between the upper and lower segments of the esophagus
                                    (8:750)

159. The most common kidney complication in the newborn child is

A. bilateral renal agenesis
B. congenital cystic kidneys
C. double kidneys
D. none of the above   (8:751)

160. Which one of the following is considered to be a possible cause of talipes in the newborn?

A. intrauterine infection
B. placental insufficiency
C. small uterine cavity
D. intrauterine position   (8:753)

161. Which of the following symptoms are associated with intracranial hemorrhage in the newborn?

1. twitchings or spasms of the whole body
2. recurring attacks of cyanosis
3. sharp, shrill, weak cry

4. grunting respirations
5. jaundice resulting from cell destruction

A. 1, 2, 3
B. 1, 4, 5
C. 2, 3, 4
D. all except 5   (4:597−8)

162. If CNS depressant medications given to a woman during labor have caused respiratory depression resulting from narcosis in the newborn, which of the following medications can be given to the infant as an antidote?

1. phenobarbital sodium
2. levallorphan (Lorfan)
3. dilantin
4. nalorphine (Nalline)

A. 1, 3
B. 3, 4
C. 1, 2
D. 2, 4   (6:292)

163. Which of the following conditions exists in male infants when the opening of the meatus is located in the dorsal shaft of the penis?

A. epispadias
B. hypospadias
C. phimosis
D. none of the above   (1:171)

164. The normal length of the testes at birth is

A. 0.5 to 1 cm
B. 1.5 to 2 cm
C. 2.5 to 3 cm
D. none of the above   (1:174)

165. Which of the following conditions is termed Klumpke's paralysis?

A. limp arm
B. lack of movement on one side of the face
C. relaxed wrist and hand, poor or absent grasp reflex
D. none of the above   (6:438)

166. In the male newborn, when the testicles are present in the inguinal canal, the condition is referred to as

A. monorchidism
B. phimosis
C. cryptorchidism
D. none of the above   (6:395)

167. Which of the following symptoms are commonly seen in the postpartum infant?

    1. pale skin
    2. absence of vernix
    3. dry, cracked skin
    4. absence of lanugo

    A. 1, 3, 4
    B. 2, 4
    C. none of the above
    D. all of the above   (6:440)

168. Impetigo in the newborn is caused by

    1. *Candida albicans*
    2. staphylococcus
    3. streptococcus
    4. *Escherichia coli*

    A. 1, 2
    B. 2, 3
    C. 2, 3, 4
    D. all of the above   (6:429)

169. The normal serum calcium level in the newborn is

    A. 2 to 4 mg/dL
    B. 5 to 7 mg/dL
    C. 8 to 10 mg/dL
    D. 11 to 12 mg/dL   (6:449)

170. Which of the following are clinical signs of hypocalcemia?

    1. high-pitched cry
    2. vomiting
    3. cyanotic periods
    4. failure to nurse well
    5. apnea

    A. 1, 2, 4
    B. 2, 3, 4
    C. 1, 3, 5
    D. none of the above   (6:449)

171. Hypocalcemia in the newborn is caused by

    A. abnormal enzyme function
    B. decreased amount of ionized calcium
    C. congenital factors
    D. none of the above   (6:449)

172. Meconium ileus is seen in approximately what percentage of newborns who later show other manifestations of fibrocystic disease?

    A. 5 to 10%
    B. 10 to 15%
    C. 15 to 20%
    D. 20 to 25%   (2:410)

173. Which of the following tests is used in partial diagnosis of fibrocystic disease?

    A. analysis of pancreatic juice for pancreatic enzymes
    B. biopsy of liver for liver enzymes
    C. saliva test
    D. none of the above   (6:455)

174. Meconium ileus is the earliest manifestation of

    A. imperforate anus
    B. tracheoesophageal fistula
    C. cystic fibrosis of the pancreas
    D. none of the above   (6:455)

175. Approximately how long does it take for nicotine to be found in the breast milk of a mother who smokes a cigarette?

    A. within four hours
    B. within six hours
    C. within eight hours
    D. nicotine is never found in breast milk   (6:419)

176. Which of the following statements best indicates the incidence of congenital heart defects in the newborn?

    A. 2 of every 100 infants
    B. 3 of every 300 infants
    C. 4 of every 500 infants
    D. 5 of every 1,000 infants   (1:131)

177. Which of the following drugs are used to treat withdrawal symptoms of infants born to addicted mothers?

    A. paregoric one to two drops per kilogram of body weight every four to six hours
    B. phenobarbital 8 mg per kilogram of body weight per day
    C. chlorpromazine 0.75 mg per kilogram of body weight every six hours
    D. all of the above   (6:440)

Directions: Each group of numbered words or phrases is followed by a list of lettered statements. MATCH the lettered statement with the numbered word or phrase most closely associated with it.

Questions 178 through 181
178. bile-stained vomitus
179. persistent vomiting
180. projectile vomiting during or immediately after feeding
181. frequent vomiting; small amounts of uncoagulated milk

A. chalasia
B. pylorospasms
C. suggestive of intestinal obstruction
D. pyloric stenosis   (6:432)

Questions 182 through 185

182. extension of infant's big toe and flexion of other toes when side of foot is stroked
183. rejection by the infant of any substance placed on the anterior portion of the tongue
184. swallowing of fluids
185. the flexing and grasping of an object placed in the palm of the infant

   A. Palmer reflex
   B. Babinski reflex
   C. deglutition reflex
   D. extrusion reflex   (6:396–7)

Questions 186 through 189

186. bilirubin level of 12 mg/dL in full-term infant
187. jaundice of nuclear masses and ganglia on the medulla
188. positive direct Coombs' with cord blood hemoglobin less than 14 g/dL for the low-birth-weight infant
189. bilirubin level, 5 to 7 mg/dL on third day

   A. kernicterus
   B. physiologic jaundice
   C. hyperbilirubinemia
   D. exchange transfusion   (6:402, 442–4)

Directions: This part of the test consists of a situation followed by a series of incomplete statements. Study the situation and select the best answer to complete each statement that follows.

Questions 190 through 201

Mrs. Kingston is a 33-year-old gravida I, Rh negative woman, who just delivered a living male infant approximately six weeks prior to her calculated date of confinement. The pregnancy was uneventful, and Mrs. Kingston was awake and participating during the labor and delivery. Observation of the infant immediately following birth reveals a healthy infant of approximately 5 lb, 14 oz who cried spontaneously.

190. Mrs. Kingston comments, "When I first saw the head coming, I thought that he was dead because the head was so blue." The nurse's best response would be

   A. "I'm sorry that you were not told of this phenomenon as part of your prenatal education."
   B. "If you hadn't been watching the delivery, you would never have noticed this phenomenon."

C. "Don't worry; everything is all right."
D. "I'm glad that you asked about this. It is a normal phenomenon that occurs in all babies."
E. none of the above   (4:343)

191. Mrs. Kingston then asks whether her son is a premature infant. The best response would probably be

   A. "Your son is less than 37 weeks of gestation; therefore he is premature."
   B. "Your son appears to weigh more than 5½ lb; therefore he is not premature."
   C. "Your son looks and appears to behave like a child who is close to term."
   D. "Your son is less than 37 weeks of gestation, and premature by this criterion. However, his body size seems to indicate that he weighs more than a premature baby."
   E. none of the above   (3:795)

192. Baby Kingston is placed in a heated crib in the delivery room. The reason for this is to prevent loss of body heat by

   A. evaporation
   B. convection
   C. conduction
   D. all of the above
   E. none of the above   (8:547–8)

193. Which one of the following observations in the umbilical cord might most likely lead the doctor to suspect congenital anomalies in Baby Kingston?

   A. true knot
   B. false knot
   C. one vein —two arteries
   D. one artery —one vein
   E. short cord   (8:406)

194. Which of the following procedures will probably be carried out in the delivery room?

   A. Apgar scoring
   B. prophylaxis against ophthalmia neonatorum
   C. infant identification
   D. all of the above
   E. none of the above   (2:172–6)

195. Mrs. Kingston requests that she be allowed to breast feed her baby while still in the delivery room. This request should be permitted because

   A. it stimulates the uterus to contract
   B. it should not be permitted

C.   the mother has colostrum in her breasts
D.   the mother has milk in her breasts
E.   the infant is hungry   (3:602)

Baby Kingston is taken to the newborn nursery. The following information was recorded on his chart: sternal retractions —muscle tone poor.

196.   Baby Kingston should be placed in

A.   a crib with his head elevated slightly
B.   a crib with his feet elevated slightly
C.   an incubator with heat control
D.   an incubator with heat and humidity controls
E.   an incubator with heat, humidity, and oxygen controls   (8:705)

197.   Baby Kingston should be watched closely for signs of

A.   erythroblastosis
B.   hypoglycemia
C.   gastrointestinal abnormalities
D.   neonatal respiratory distress syndrome
E.   none of the above   (8:701)

198.   Which of the following would probably indicate that Baby Kingston had hyaline membrane disease?

A.   chest retractions within the first hour of life
B.   granular appearance and presence of air in the bronchi (seen on x-ray)
C.   respiratory rate over 60/min within a few hours after birth
D.   all of the above
E.   none of the above   (8:704)

199.   Baby Kingston was started on

A.   feedings of glucose through a nipple
B.   feedings of glucose via the intravenous route
C.   feedings of glucose and sodium bicarbonate via the intravenous route
D.   feedings of formula through a nipple
E.   breast feeding   (8:707)

200.   By the fourth day of life, Baby Kingston's condition was greatly improved. This was most probably due to

A.   intake of glucose over a period of time
B.   the production of surfactant within the child's lungs
C.   oxygen therapy
D.   the stabilizing of the child's body temperature
E.   none of the above   (8:704)

201.   Baby Kingston's chances for survival after the fourth day were

A.   minimal
B.   poor
C.   fair
D.   good
E.   excellent   (8:704)

Questions 202 through 215
Baby Boy Lang has just been admitted to the nursery. The delivery room record indicates that his mother "fell" three days ago and that she was admitted to the labor room this morning with "bleeding." Baby Boy Lang was born spontaneously following a two-hour labor. His Apgar scores are 5 and 7, his weight is 3 lb, 10 oz, and he is immediately placed in an incubator with oxygen and humidity.

202.   Baby Lang is approximately how premature, using his weight as the criterion?

A.   4 weeks
B.   6 weeks
C.   8 weeks
D.   10 weeks   (8:103−4)

203.   Baby Lang has a greater predisposition to heat loss than a full-term infant for which of the following reasons?

A.   poor metabolic response to cold
B.   decreased activity
C.   low thermal stability
D.   all of the above   (6:470−1)

204.   Baby Lang should be dressed in which of the following ways?

A.   diaper
B.   diaper and shirt
C.   diaper, shirt, and wrapped in a blanket
D.   he should not be dressed at all   (3:773−4)

205.   Baby Lang's temperature should be maintained at

A.   96°F
B.   97°F
C.   98.6°F
D.   99.0°F   (6:471)

206.   Which of the following would probably be present in Baby Lang?

1.   weak grasp reflex
2.   skull bone cartilaginous
3.   silky hair on the head
4.   undescended testicles
5.   transverse creases on soles of feet

A. 1, 2, 4
B. 1, 3, 5
C. all of the above
D. none of the above (6:468)

207. Baby Lang should be placed in which of the following positions in the incubator?

A. on his abdomen with his head turned to one side or the other
B. on his back with head and shoulders elevated with a small, rolled blanket
C. on his back with head and shoulders flat
D. none of the above (3:776)

208. If Baby Lang displays a weak sucking reflex he will probably be fed

A. intravenously
B. by nasogastric tube
C. with a premie nipple
D. with a duck bill nipple (6:474)

209. Baby Lang will not be fed for approximately 12 to 24 hours. Then he will probably receive a first feeding of

A. 2 mL of glucose and water
B. 5 mL of glucose and water
C. 8 mL of glucose and water
D. 10 mL of glucose and water (8:676)

210. The caloric needs of Baby Lang are now much greater than those of a full-term infant. They are

A. 10 to 20% per pound of body weight
B. 15 to 20% per pound of body weight
C. 30 to 50% per pound of body weight
D. none of the above (6:474)

211. Jaundice in Baby Lang can be expected

A. within the first 24 hours
B. during the second to the fourth days
C. between the fourth and fifth days
D. jaundice is not expected to occur in Baby Lang (3:802)

212. The incidence of prematurity is higher in which of the following?

1. mothers under the age of 16
2. multigravidas over the age of 40
3. plural births
4. cigarette-smoking mothers
5. middle-class mothers

A. 1, 2, 4
B. 1, 3, 4
C. 2, 3, 4
D. all of the above (6:466–7)

213. Which of the following contribute(s) to infant mortality?

A. maternal age
B. spacing of children
C. low birth weight
D. all of the above (6:469)

214. Mrs. Lang's first response to her baby boy will probably be

1. grief
2. preparation for his death
3. hope for his survival
4. depression
5. first attempts at forming a relationship

A. 1, 4, 5
B. 2, 3
C. 1, 5
D. all of the above (3:805–6)

215. Which of the following complications might arise in Baby Lang's

1. Mikity-Wilson syndrome
2. hypoglycemia
3. hyaline membrane disease
4. retrolental fibroplasia

A. 1, 2, 4
B. 1, 3, 4
C. 2, 3, 4
D. all of the above (6:479–87)

Answers and Explanations:
The Newborn

1. **C.** Thus, viability occurs at about the twenty-sixth week of gestation, that is, when the lungs are mature enough to allow for maintenance of lung expansion and exchange of gases.

2. **B.** Respiration usually is established within one minute after birth and is accompanied by a lusty cry.

3. **C.** If surfactant is not present, the surface tension of the lungs is more difficult to overcome. An adequate supply of surfactant does not seem to be available in both the premature and immature baby. This is thought to be a contributing cause of hyaline membrane disease.

4. **B.** The main component of surfactant is lecithin.

5. **D.** High-pressure oxygen can severely damage the alvelar cells, which produce surfactant. Chilling of the baby after birth may result in a reduction of available oxygen and glucose, produce acidosis, and result in a decrease in circulation that inhibits the production of surfactant. The lungs of the immature baby do not produce adequate amounts of surfactant.

6. **C.** The infant's airway must be clear in order to establish respiration and prevent aspiration.

7. **D.** The exact mechanism by which the respirations are initiated is not known.

8. **D.** At present, the majority of obstetricians appear to favor early rather than late clamping of the cord.

9. **C.** Apgar scoring system is based on five signs, that of heart rate, respiration effort, muscle tone, reflex irritability, and color. Each sign is given a score of 0, 1, or 2. Scores of each of the signs are added together for a maximum score of 10.

10. **D.** The highest score a newborn can receive on any five signs is 2.

11. **A.** Silver nitrate 1%, or penicillin ophthalmic ointment, will destroy the causative organism, *Neisseria gonorrhoeae*.

12. **B.** The usual dosage of vitamin K is 1.0 mg.

13. **D.** All of the above-mentioned factors contribute to the relative instability of the newborn's body temperature.

14. **C.** The circulation at this time has characteristics that are neither those of a fetal nor an adult pattern. This transition to adult circulation is usually complete in several days.

15. **D.** All the above-mentioned factors lead to the establishment of the adult pattern of circulation.

16. **D.** Although the transition from fetal to adult pattern of circulation is usually complete in a few days, anatomic occlusion of fetal vessels is not complete for weeks or months.

17. **A.** The greatest mortality rate of any period of infancy and childhood occurs during this period. Thus, it is an important time span for study.

18. **B.** There are, however, wide variations in birth weights of normal full-term infants.

19. **D.** The usual range is between 18 and 25 in.

20. **A.** This position is usually one of symmetry, with limbs semiflexed and hips slightly abducted.

21. **B.** In babies born in vertex position, this can be a sign of hypotonia, or floppy infant syndrome.

22. **B.** The head constitutes about one fourth of the total body weight.

23. **A.** The skull bones are not united but can overlap during labor and delivery.

24. **A.** The head circumference is about 2 cm greater than the chest measurement at birth.

25. **B.** Smegma is the name given to the substance which is found between the folds of the labia.

26. **B.** The sebaceous glands become quiescent shortly after birth because of the absence of maternal androgens. They become active again at puberty.

27. **A.** These hemangiomas are clusters of small capillaries.

28. **C.** The mature infant has many creases criss-crossing the entire sole of the foot. The immature infant has fewer creases running along the length of the sole.

29. **B.** It is triangular in shape and may be almost closed at birth.

30. **B.** Cephalhematoma gradually becomes larger until about the seventh day of life; it remains stationary for a time and then begins to subside.

31. **B.** The sluggish peripheral circulation accounts for the blueness of the newborn's hands and feet.

32. **D.** Lanugo is the fine hair found over the newborn's body. Milia are small sebaceous cysts found on the child's nose. Mongolian spots are blue-black discolorations seen on the buttocks, back, and sacral regions of white babies from dark parents.

33. **B.** The cause is not known. It disappears without treatment.

34. **B.** The color of the eyes changes from blue to its permanent color at about the sixth month of age.

35. **C.** The child's vision is not as acute as the adult's. However, a certain amount of visual differentiation is possible for them.

36. **C.** Acute hearing occurs within several days.

37. **B.** Rate and rhythm of respirations can be easily altered by stimuli and may vary with activity.

38. **B.** There is much variability in the pulse rate of the newborn, with a high of 170 beats during crying and a low of between 80 and 90 beats during sleep.

39. **A.** The average number of red blood cells in the normal newborn at birth is 5 million per cubic mm, with a range of 4 million to 6 million.

40. **C.** Polymorphonuclear cells account for a large percentage of the total count.

41. **D.** The blood in the newborn may account for about 10% of the body weight.

42. **D.** Meconium begins to form in the intestine by the end of the fourth month.

43. **C.** They appear between the third and fifth days of life.

44. **A.** By the end of a week the newborn voids approximately 7 oz per day.

45. **B.** The engorged breasts may secrete "witches milk," which, without interference, will disappear spontaneously.

46. **B.** The temperature of the newborn returns to normal in approximately 8 hours following birth.

47. **C.** Approximately 70 to 75% of the total body weight of the newborn is extracellular water.

48. **C.** The normal bleeding time in the newborn is two minutes.

49. **C.** The normal coagulation time in the newborn is three minutes.

50. **A.** Other contraindications for circumcision include an abnormal coagulation time and clinical manifestations of jaundice.

51. **A.** The prothrombin level is highest at birth, then declines until the eighth day when it again reaches normal levels.

52. **C.** The hemoglobin level at birth measures from 14 to 19 g/dL of blood.

53. **C.** A level above 13 mg/dL of blood is considered above a physiologic value.

54. **B.** This decrease in body weight is caused by a loss of excess fluid from the body tissues and the low fluid intake of the infant.

55. **D.** It is difficult to estimate the capacity of the stomach, since the feedings may empty into the duodenum even before the feeding is complete.

56. **A.** The yawn reflex draws in additional oxygen.

57. **C.** The salivary glands are immature at birth and produce little saliva until the child is about three months old.

58. **C.** The peak incidence of the tonic neck reflex is at about two to three months. Constant display of this behavior, particularly before two or three months of age, may indicate problems in achieving developmental stages.

59. **B.** The response may have to be repeated several times for the examiner to be able to observe all components.

60. **D.** Absence of moro reflex during first four to five months indicates possible problems for the newborn.

61. **C.** These reflexes are responsible for getting food to the stomach. They are active in full-term infants but may be absent in the premature infant.

62. **D.** Answer 2 is partially correct; skin erythema is normal; however, newborn stools should not be loose.

63. **C.** These raised areas appear during the first or second month of life and the majority of these hemangiomas disappear when the child is between the ages of seven and eight.

64. **B.** The frenulum linguae sometimes extends to the tip of the tongue. In such cases, the doctor may cut the tip of the frenulum.

65. **D.** Tearing in the newborn may be due to the blockage of the lacrimal ducts by exudate resulting from the irritation of silver nitrate.

66. **A.** Pregnanediol, which is an excretion product of progesterone, is found in human breast milk and inhibits the activity of glucuronyl transferase.

67. **A.** In physiologic jaundice, the Coombs' test is negative.

68. **C.** Bilirubin is released during the destruction of red blood cells. The inability of the liver to remove the bilirubin from the blood results in the jaundice.

69. **A.** When the bilirubin level goes above 12 mg/dL, the full-term infant is said to have hyperbilirubinemia.

70. **D.** The liver enzyme, glucuronyl transferase, is responsible for the conversion of the insoluble form of bilirubin to a soluble form so that it can be excreted by the liver into the intestines and by the kidneys into the urine.

71. **B.** In the breast-fed infant, the inoffensive odor is the result of fermentation, and there are frequent movements because of the ease with which feces pass through the colon.

72. **B.** The *Lactobacillus bifidus* act upon the lactose and convert it into lactic acid.

73. **D.** The high lactose content facilitates amino acid, calcium, phosphorus, and magnesium absorption, and nitrogen retention. Thus, mineral content of the bones is increased. The *Lactobacillus bifidus* convert the lactose into lactic acid, which in turn hinders growth of pathogens. The production of riboflavin and pyridoxine is favored when lactose is the principal carbohydrate in milk.

74. **D.** The protein is acted upon by the gastric chemistry, pancreatic and intestinal secretions.

75. **D.** Digital examination stimulates peristalsis and contributes to spontaneous passage of the mass.

76. **C.** Bowel movements following each feeding are the result of gastrocolic reflex. As the food enters the stomach, it stimulates peristalsis in the lower intestinal tract.

77. **C.** Miliaria is prickly heat, and the most frequent cause is that of overdressing the baby.

78. **C.** Seborrheic dermatitis is "cradle cap" and is described as a red macular rash that starts on the forehead and then spreads to the cheeks, neck, and chest.

79. **A.** The mother should be encouraged to wash and rinse the scalp, particularly the area over the soft spot, daily with soap and water.

80. **C.** A mild diaper rash is best described as erythematous nonraised areas spread over the genital and buttock area.

81. **A.** Epstein's pearls are found along the alveolar ridge or bilaterally along the median raphe. They are accumulations of epithelial cells and are white, glistening, circular patches.

82. **D.** All of the factors mentioned can contribute to functional vomiting in the newborn.

83. **B.** The recommended amount of protein for the normal newborn is 0.9 to 1.4 grams per pound of body weight per day.

84. **B.** An iron intake of 1 to 2 mg/kg of body weight is the recommended daily amount.

85. **B.** The infant probably needs to have a stronger formula if it cries an hour or so following a feeding and takes large amounts of formula at frequent intervals.

86. **B.** Colostrum has a higher amount of protein than does milk.

87. **D.** Caloric needs vary a great deal even for infants of the same size and weight. Activity seems to be a determining factor.

88. **C.** Because the surface area of the newborn is large in comparison with his weight.

89. **D.** All the factors must be taken into account when determining the caloric intake for the child during the neonatal period.

90. **C.** Or 50 to 55 calories per pound per day.

91. **B.** Or 50 to 60 calories per pound per day.

92. **D.** It is caused by a low fluid intake during the first days of life and the usual fluid loss that occurs in the immediate postnatal period.

93. **A.** The fever and side effects can be taken care of by increasing oral feedings.

94. **C.** Essentially this means that the interval between feedings may vary from two to eight hours.

95. **A.** Infants have a relatively large percentage of body fluid, but their ability to withstand an inadequate fluid intake is not as efficient as that of an older child or adult. An adequate amount of fluid intake is essential.

96. **C.** Or 2⅓ to 3 oz per lb of body weight per 24 hours.

97. **D.** This is 1.2 to 1.5 oz per lb of body weight per 24 hours.

98. **D.** All of the factors mentioned influence the method of choice in infant feeding.

99. **B.** These sinuses lie just behind and beneath the areolar part of the breast.

100. **A.** Colostrum is produced by the secretory activity of the alveolar cells. Colostrum is present until about the third day after delivery, when milk production starts.

101. **C.** Studies have shown that the child whose needs are met quickly and consistently soon realizes that he can trust others to come as soon as he signals, without having to make his needs known by crying.

102. **C.** Following the feeding, the child will again sleep for several hours, awakening only when uncomfortable because of hunger or a wet diaper.

103. **B.** In the mild cases, there is cyanosis of the entire body, and muscle tone is good. This condition is called *asphyxia livida*. In the more severe cases, the infant has marked pallor and poor muscle tone. This is known as *asphyxia pallida*.

104. **D.** Intrauterine hypoxia, drugs, and central nervous system trauma are the three major causes of failure of the infant to breathe at birth or failure of the infant to establish adequate respiration.

105. **A.** The greatest incidence of hyaline membrane disease is seen in the infant between 1,000 and 1,500 g, and it is seen in about 10% of all premature infants.

106. **D.** It is known that the hyaline membrane is a protein; the cause of its formation is not absolutely known.

107. **D.** Expiratory grunting may be the earliest sign of the disease, and cessation of expiratory grunting is often the first sign of improvement.

108. **D.** It is prone to happen in the prolonged labor of the primipara where there may be difficult forceps deliveries, lesions, or extractions.

109. **D.** Signs of intracranial injury may be generalized and similar to those produced by respiratory distress and congenital heart disease.

110. **D.** In addition, the child who has cerebral injury may have irregular respirations, cyanosis at intervals or continuously, failure to nurse well, and forceful vomiting.

111. **C.** With cerebral injury the moro reflex is often present for several days after birth. It then disppears and returns much later.

112. **C.** Rest and quiet may inhibit the amount of intracranial bleeding. The child is handled only when necessary.

113. **B.** The raising of the head is believed to reduce intracranial pressure.

114. **D.** The child is usually placed in an incubator where he can receive warmth and oxygen as needed. Vitamin K may decrease the amount of bleeding by preventing the transitory defect in blood coagulation that occurs in the early neonatal period. Phenobarbital 1/8 g (given two to four times a day) may be used for sedation.

115. **B.** Cerebral palsy is also caused by congenital defects and by other postnatal conditions such as erythroblastosis, asphyxia, and head injuries.

116. **D.** Everyone who is in contact with infants should assume this responsibility, both parents and personnel.

117. **A.** This organism is found in the genital tract of the woman and can be transmitted to the child during birth.

118. **D.** The causative organism, *Neisseria gonorrhoroeae*, can be found in the genital canal of infected women and can also be transmitted by personnel and articles that come in contact with the organism.

119. **B.** Irritation from the silver nitrate drops is present only during the first day of life. Gonorrheal conjunctivitis appears within two to three days after birth.

120. **C.** The spirochetes are transmitted from the mother to the infant through the placenta sometime between the fifth month of pregnancy and the end of pregnancy.

121. **D.** The serologic test for syphilis becomes positive after several months when the infant develops antibodies in its own blood.

122. **B.** Hemolytic disease of the newborn can result from any blood group incompatibility. Edema is usually seen only in stillborn infants or in those who die shortly after birth.

123. **A.** Rh incompatibility usually arises when an Rh negative woman is carrying an Rh positive fetus.

124. **D.** In the individual baby, any one of the three factors mentioned may predominate.

125. **C.** RhoGAM is a prepared gamma globulin that contains a concentration of Rh antibodies.

126. **B.** If the man is heterozygous positive he will have one positive gene (D) and one negative gene

(d) for the Rh factor. Thus, there is a 50-50 chance of the couple having an Rh negative baby.

127. **D.** The umbilical cord blood is positive when there are anti-Rh antibodies in the baby's blood system even when there is absence of clinical evidence of the disease.

128. **B.** The infant of a diabetic mother suffers from an excessive lowering of blood glucose because of the large amount of circulating insulin. As liver glycogen is broken down to elevate the baby's blood glucose level, the elevation of the glucose level causes more secreting of insulin, resulting in still greater hypoglycemia.

129. **B.** Hyaline membrane disease occurs in about 50% of all infants of diabetic mothers.

130. **D.** All of the factors mentioned have been shown to contribute to congenital abnormality in the newborn infant.

131. **B.** Prefix hydro means of or having to do with water, and cephalic means in the head.

132. **D.** The esophagus ends in a blind pouch rather than a continuous tube to the stomach.

133. **D.** The exact cause is not known.

134. **B.** It is seen more frequently in female infants.

135. **C.** Incomplete fusion of maxillary or pre-maxillary processes and the palatal processes results in cleft lip or cleft palate.

136. **C.** Because of the connection existing between the mouth and nose in a baby with a cleft palate, milk taken via the mouth will come out of the nose unless careful feeding techniques are carried out. This connection also contributes to respiratory infections.

137. **D.** Cleft lip is a fissure of the upper lip to the side of the midline and may vary from a slight notch to a complete separation.

138. **D.** Here, an extra chromosome belonging to either pair 21 or 22 or a translocation of 15/21 is present.

139. **B.** Other characteristics of Down's syndrome include protruding tongue, underdeveloped muscles, loose joints, and heart and alimentary tract abnormalities.

140. **C.** Advanced maternal age appears to a major factor in the etiology of this disorder.

141. **B.** Formerly, a birth weight of 2,500 g or less was considered to be the determining criterion. Now, however, the use of weight as the sole criteria for evaluation of a premature infant is felt to be inadequate.

142. **B.** The term "low birth weight" infant has now replaced the term "premature."

143. **D.** All factors mentioned are considered to be causes of death in the immature baby.

144. **D.** Maternal factors include such things as toxemia, placenta abruptio, age, and parity. Paternal factors may possibly include factors such as elderly age, transmission of Rh positive genes, and diabetes mellitus. Among those listed under placental factors, placental insufficiency and cord abnormalities have been listed.

145. **D.** All statements are true. They may vary in infants of approximately the same size, depending on the factors associated with prematurity and the physical condition of mother and infant.

146. **A.** Recent studies indicate that premature infants do well when the relative humidity in the incubator is kep between 40 and 60%.

147. **A.** Infants with RDS tend to develop hyperbilirubinemia because of delayed functioning of their enzyme system.

148. **B.** The largest number of inborn errors of metabolism are autosomal-recessive disorders.

149. **B.** Phenylalanine hydroxylase is necessary to change phenylalanine into tyrosine.

150. **D.** The child with PKU is usually normal at birth but without treatment usually becomes severely retarded.

151. **C.** Blood levels of phenylalanine have reached as high as 60 mg/dL.

152. **D.** This diet should be started as soon as possible. Commercial products such as Lofenlac are available.

153. **C.** The blood test is done routinely on all babies in the nursery.

154. **B.** Peripheral nerve injuries occur during birth.

155. **B.** Facial paralysis may occur as a result of pressure on the facial nerve during labor or from the forceps blade during delivery.

156. **A.** Injury to the fifth and sixth cervical nerves results from forcible pulling of the shoulder away from the head during delivery, usually during a breech extraction.

157. **C.** The clavicle can be broken during an easy delivery or during a difficult delivery at the infant's shoulders.

158. **C.** There is hypertrophy of the musculature of the pylorus, chiefly of the circular muscles, which in turn constrict the lumen of the pyloric opening.

159. **B.** There are present in the kidneys both large and small cysts, which may not cause problems for several years or until adulthood. Kidney function will eventually become impaired.

160. **D.** Talipes, or clubfoot, is a deformity in which an unequal pull of muscles forces the foot to be held at an abnormal angle. It has been attributed to intrauterine position or muscular imbalance.

161. **D.** All of the symptoms mentioned except jaundice are associated with intracranial hemorrhage.

162. **D.** Both nalorphine (Nalline) and levallorphan (Lorfan) relieve respiratory depression caused by narcotics. Dosage is 0.25 mg into the umbilical vein.

163. **A.** The condition known as epispadias exists when the opening of the urinary meatus is located on the dorsal shaft of the penis.

164. **B.** The normal length of the penis at birth is 1.5 to 2 cm. The size of the penis begins to increase at the age of eleven.

165. **C.** Klumpke's paralysis, a form of brachial palsy, results from damage to the eighth cervical and first thoracic nerve roots.

166. **C.** When the testicles remain in the inguinal canal following birth, the condition is referred to as cryptorchidism.

167. **D.** The postmature infant is one born after the forty-second week of gestation. He does not have to be a victim of placental dysfunction. Thus, symptoms associated with placental dysfunction need not be present.

168. **B.** Impetigo in the newborn is caused by staphylococcus or streptococcus.

169. **C.** The normal serum calcium level in the newborn is 8 to 10 mg/dL.

170. **C.** The clinical signs of hypocalcemia are also common in other disorders.

171. **B.** Hypocalcemia is treated with 10% calcium gluconate, usually in doses of 1 to 1.5 mg per kg of body weight, given intravenously.

172. **A.** The lack of sufficient pancreatic enzymes before birth results in impaired digestive activity. The meconium becomes viscid and causes an obstruction in the small intestines.

173. **A.** An analysis of pancreatic juices will show an absence of pancreatic enzymes in the child who has cystic fibrosis.

174. **C.** Meconium ileus is the earliest manifestation of cystic fibrosis of the pancreas.

175. **A.** Nicotine is found in breast milk within four hours following smoking.

176. **D.** About five in every thousand infants are born with a congenital heart defect.

177. **D.** All of the drugs mentioned are used to treat the withdrawal symptoms of infants born to addicted mothers.

178. **C.** The vomiting of bile-stained substances is suggestive of intestinal obstruction.

179. **B.** Persistent vomiting is suggestive of pylorospasms.

180. **D.** Projectile vomiting is characteristic of pyloric stenosis.

181. **A.** Frequent vomiting of small amounts of uncoagulated milk indicates chalasia, an abnormally relayed esophageal muscle.

182. **B.** Babinski's reflex is elicited when the side of the infant's foot is stroked.

183. **D.** Extrusion reflex causes the infant to reject any substance placed on the anterior portion of the tongue.

184. **C.** Deglutition reflex causes the infant to swallow fluids.

185. **A.** Palmer reflex occurs when a small object is placed in the palm of the infant's hand.

186. **C.** Hyperbilirubinemia is present in the normal newborn when the bilirubin level reaches 12 mg/dL.

187. **A.** Kernicterus is defined as jaundice of nuclear masses and ganglia on the medulla.

188. **D.** An exchange transfusion is indicated when there is a positive direct Coombs' test and the cord blood hemoglobin is less than 14 g/dL in the low-birth-weight infant.

189. **B.** Physiologic jaundice can be defined as a bilirubin level of 5 to 7 mg/dL on the third day.

190. **D.** Cyanosis is present in all babies at birth. As the infant's circulation changes from the fetal pattern to one of extrauterine life and he breathes, the skin becomes pink.

191. **C.** The premature or immature infant should be identified by evaluation of his weight and gestational age. In evaluating this gestational age, the history of the mother's last menstrual period is of great importance.

192. **D.** All of the factors mentioned. The child loses body heat with the *evaporation* of amniotic fluid from his body. The child may lose heat by *convection* when the warmth from his body flows to the cool air in the delivery room. He may also lose heat by *conduction* when the heat from his body flows to the cool sheet on which he is placed for care.

193. **D.** Infants with only one umbilical artery are reported to have a higher incidence of congenital anomalies, especially renal and gastrointestinal.

194. **D.** All of the above-mentioned procedures.

195. **A.** Nursing stimulates the pituitary gland to secrete oxytocin.

196. **E.** Baby Kingston should be placed in an incubator where his total environment can be controlled.

197. **D.** Babies who are immature at birth are very susceptible to the neonatal respiratory distress syndrome (hyaline membrane disease).

198. **D.** All of the factors mentioned are important in helping to establish a diagnosis of hyaline membrane disease.

199. **C.** Glucose solution is given early in life to provide adequate nutrition and insure a satisfactory blood sugar level. Sodium bicarbonate is given to correct the disturbance in the acid-base balance of the blood.

200. **B.** The production of pulmonary surfactant that occurs within 12 to 48 hours assists the alveoli to become aerated and the atelectasis disappears. The child thus breathes more easily, and recovery occurs.

201. **E.** Once the production of pulmonary surfactant starts, the child is well on his way to recovery.

202. **C.** Using weight as the criteria for determining the degree of maturity, it would be assumed that Baby Lang was born close to the end of the eighth month of development.

203. **D.** All of the factors mentioned contribute to the premature infant's predisposition to heat loss.

204. **D.** Baby Lang should be left undressed so that the warm air will have direct contact with his body.

205. **B.** Once Baby Lang's temperature reaches 97°F, the incubator temperature should be adjusted to meet his needs.

206. **A.** In the premature infant, the hair on the head will be fuzzy, and the soles of the feet are almost smooth and almost without creases.

207. **B.** Baby Lang should be placed on his back with his head and shoulders extended. Also, the arms should be kept flexed and abducted and away from the chest. This will permit greater expansion of the thoracic area.

208. **B.** It is generally agreed that a child who weighs over 3½ lb should be fed by nasogastric tube if it has a weak sucking and swallowing reflex.

209. **B.** Baby Lang will probably receive a first feeding of glucose and water, depending on his ability to tolerate this.

210. **C.** Baby Lang's caloric needs are 30 to 50% greater per pound of body weight than those of a full-term infant.

211. **B.** The immature liver is unable to conjugate the bilirubin created by the red blood cell breakdown.

212. **B.** Studies also show that women who receive care through clinics are more likely to deliver low-birth-weight and premature infants. This is attributed to the low socioeconomic status of the clinic patient.

213. **D.** Infants in the low-birth-weight category approximate 10% of live births, and the mortality among neonates is generally directly proportional to the number of infants born with weights less than 2,500 g.

214. **B.** Following the birth of a premature infant, the mother experiences anticipatory grief. She withdraws from the relationship she formed with the child during pregnancy. She hopes that her child will live but at the same time prepares herself for his possible death.

215. **D.** All of the complications mentioned are seen in the premature infant. The Mikity-Wilson syndrome is a respiratory disorder that occurs during the third week of life. The premature infant's blood sugar concentration at birth ranges from 20 to 100 mg/dL. Retrolental fibroplasia can occur in premature infants, regardless of whether the child has received oxygen or not. Hyaline membrane disease is a respiratory distress syndrome that, among other features, is more common in male infants.